Intermittent Fasting For Women 101

The Essentials and 30 Day Challenge For Proven Weight Loss Results

Wing Horse Media Circles

Will Ramos & Gin Fung

Contents:

For the horses

My other books

Chapter 1:
Introduction

I want to admit something to you, dear reader, right up front.

When I first heard that fasting could be an amazing, natural, and healthy way to lose weight and have a healthy lifestyle, I shuddered. All I could picture was the times I myself had been ravenously hungry ('hangry', right?). It wasn't exactly appealing.

But when I realized that it wasn't about starving myself for hours and hours on end and it was more about using fasting times to lose weight, I became intrigued.

I became even more intrigued when the weight started to drop off.

That started me on an incredible journey. It's a journey that I will share with you in multiple ways throughout this entire book.

It's not a physical journey. I didn't start in New York and ended up in California. No, not at all. I started in an unhealthy, overweight body and then I kept trying the fasting times each day. I made that journey to the destination where I am today:

My extra weight is gone. I look great. Do you know how it feels to stand in front of a mirror and say to yourself, "I look great"? If you had asked me to do that two years ago, I would have cried because I was so unhappy.

Not any longer.

Girls Only Wanted!

This book was written for women, by a woman! You won't receive advice that is better suited for men. You know why?

Well, they have a completely different body than you do! A male physicality just isn't the same as a female physicality. I'm not just talking the obvious differences here.

Our women's bodies were designed to create and grow beautiful babies, and that means massive differences in our basic physiology. Our cells function differently, our organs function differently, and our entire metabolism processes nutrients differently. We're not male, and so that means big changes from male dieting and fasting advice.

You've probably seen this yourself in the real world. You try to set the same weight loss goals as a boyfriend or husband, only to watch them effortlessly lose weight just by cutting out cheeseburgers! Meanwhile, your stubborn weight doesn't budge. You're cutting out one hundred calories per day, and you're spending your thirty minutes three times a week at the gym. But nothing is happening! What's up with that? It's completely frustrating and demoralizing.

Well, in this book, I'm going to walk you through the exact female only biological processes that are going on in your cells. I want to give you real scientific answers as to why it's more difficult for you to lose weight. We'll delve right down into the cellular level and examine what's going on every time you reach for the next bite.

Forget the male Intermittent Fasting and dieting advice. This book is for women only, and I'll peel back the curtain to show you the reality of what's going on in your body.

Once you have those scientific answers, then we will work together to craft a fasting and feeding schedule that takes advantage of your body! We will work with what we've got and stop trying to make you into something you're not. Bypass that advice and choose this book instead. It's Really All

About Eating

This book is about Intermittent Fasting for women – but we're also going to spend the vast majority of this book talking about food, too! That's because in between your fasting cycles, you've gotta eat, girl.

But as soon as I mention food, dozens of questions pop up in your mind:

- What am I supposed to be eating to help me lose weight?
- What foods burn fat the fastest?
- What are the most delicious foods to help me lose weight?
- What are the 'no no' foods I can't eat?
- What am I allowed to eat while fasting? Or is it just water?
- How many calories should I eat each day?
- What kinds of calories should I be eating?
- How can I fit my meals into my busy life?
- What's the relationship between Intermittent Fasting and food?
- How many meals should I be eating?
- When should I be eating my meals?
- How big are the portion sizes that I'm allowed?
- Is it okay to be vegetarian or vegan and still do this Intermittent Fasting?
- What if I get hungry?
- Is it okay to try it for just a few days out of each week?
- How do I keep my blood sugar levels up?
- How do I know if I'm burning fat and this is working?

Yep, it really is a lot about eating. You are going to find every single answer to these questions – and more – inside this book. I have covered this food topic in-depth, especially in Chapter 4. That's because eating is such a huge part of any diet plan. Even when Intermittently Fasting, you have got to eat the right foods.

I'll also talk about exactly what you can eat during your fasting times. Yes, you can have some calories, but they have to be the right calories at the right times. We'll go into that, too!

Follow Me Step by Step

So, Intermittent Fasting is about abstaining from eating in order to lose weight and burn fat.

Okay.

But, where do you start?

You need some massive help – and this book will lay it all out for you in easy, practical steps. There are no abstract theories or vague advice present here. I live in the real world, and so do you!

You are a busy woman. You have a full work load of at least forty hours a week, you have your family with your husband and kids, you have to grocery shop, you are probably helping out with chores around the house, and many of you have added responsibilities like taking care of elderly parents, being involved with local organizations, and trying to squeeze in a little time to yourself. Not to mention fun times with friends and going out!

How in the world are you supposed to Intermittently Fast, eat the right way, and have this busy life all at the same time?

I had those exact same questions, too. Which is why when I embarked on my own Intermittent Fasting journey, I made sure to track every single little thing I was doing. In the beginning, I made plenty of mistakes, I didn't feel as good on a daily basis as I did later, and I goofed up a lot. I was also held back by my lack of knowledge about what exactly was going on in my body. I had no idea what I was doing!

But you will!

Just follow this book step by step, and you will get my results, but in a lot faster, more efficient, less time-wasting, and more informed way. That is such a relief, isn't it? Knowledge really is power. Once you have the correct knowledge about Intermittent Fasting and eating, you can rocket right to the top and achieve those weight loss goals that have been so elusive in the past.

A Brief Introduction ...

Hello, and thanks for reading about Intermittent Fasting. My name is Will Ramos, but I'm not the main author of this book! I'm just here to introduce the amazingly talented, beautiful, and successful Gin Fung. She's your Intermittent Fasting success story.

But before I do, I wanted to share my own diet, weight loss, fitness, and health story with you. Yes, I'm a man! But that does not mean I don't know the frustrations of struggling to have the body you want.

There are so many hidden carbohydrates (including all kinds of sugars) lurking in the foods you eat, that even someone who appears healthy on the outside can suffer from unexpected and severe health problems on the inside.

That's exactly what happened to me. I was a hale and healthy male athlete in my teens! I was playing sports, getting outside a lot, didn't carry any extra weight, and my BMI was totally normal. If you saw me, you'd have no idea that I was secretly unhealthy. I sure didn't know.

So, imagine my total surprise when I was suddenly diagnosed with diabetes.

Wait, what?

Yeah, whatever stereotypes you think about the average diabetes sufferer, that surely wasn't me. But suddenly, it was. I now had a disease that radically changed my relationship with food. I'd always exercised frequently, that I just didn't think it was necessary or important to care about what was on the plate. I just burned all those calories, anyway.

But diabetes has nothing to do with calories, being thin, exercising, or sports. That was eye-opening. I was thrown for a loop and struggled with my life into my early adulthood, trying everything I could think of to lessen my symptoms and get my diabetes under control. It took longer than I want to admit (especially to you!) to finally realize there was this incredible link between diet and health. Hey, I was a teenager okay?

Yet, once I recognized this link, my whole outlook changed immediately. I started with the Atkins Diet, which was popular at the time, then shortly thereafter started exploring the Keto Diet. This was around the early 2000s. The Ketogenic Diet sounded weird and extreme to me, with its ridiculously high fat contents and ridiculously low carb contents, but hey – I was already experimenting, so why not?

Well, needless to say, that Keto Diet experiment turned into a full tilt obsession as soon as my diabetes numbers started looking healthier. The more I ate this diet, the better my numbers got. Each doctor visit I was improving. I read everything I could get my hands on, including all about the nutrition, the science, the practical application, the recipes, and the meal plans. I absorbed this knowledge even better than a sponge, because my own health was at stake!

My experiments and personal field tested knowledge paid off. You might not believe me, but it's the truth:

The diabetes is gone. A long gone memory by this point.

And, I've been on the Ketogenic Diet for fourteen years.

I changed the metabolic process in my own body, I'm in ketosis 100% of the time, and I've never been healthier. On the inside and the outside this time. That was my story, and I am happy to say that it could be yours too. But wait! I see your furrowed brows. Isn't this about intermittent fasting for women, by a woman? Indeed!

So, let me introduce the real author of this book. She is the awesome superwoman hero who has put her heart and soul into this book, just so she can share it with you!

Learning From Gin's Story

Thank you, Will! Yes, my name is Gin Fung. I'm definitely a woman. Nice to meet you! I tried Intermittent Fasting for the first time five years ago, with little success. I thought it was okay, but it certainly didn't live up to the hype that several of my close girlfriends kept trying to convince me was the latest thing! I'm a skeptical person by nature. I did do the Intermittent Fasting for just a month, but I did not plan for it, I didn't commit to it, and I was mostly half-heartedly doing it just to lose a few pounds.

Needless to say, I didn't do well at all! Of course, then I thought to myself, "Oh, this whole Intermittent Fasting thing doesn't work. You just starve yourself and you're supposed to lose weight. But it didn't for me, so it doesn't work."

That was my take away from it. Until, about eight months later, I went on a dieting retreat. And, what do you know? A main portion of the retreat incorporated Intermittent Fasting. After just a week of doing it – and doing it right this time – I was shocked at the changes. I felt more energy, my basic body energy was stabilized, I felt slimmer, my clothes fit looser, and I just didn't feel as heavy, sluggish, or bloated.

Inspired, I came home and this time, I did it right! I planned for my eating windows in between fasting times, I ate the foods I was supposed to, I had my meals at the same time each day, I tracked my results ... and the weight loss was actually pretty effortless after that. Yes, I said effortless! I was so focused on the eating aspect that I didn't really feel hungry or deprived during the fasting times. It helps that my life is busy – as is yours, too!

The longer I was on Intermittent Fasting, the more results I experienced. As my energy increased and my weight loss started to escalate as the weeks went by, I embarked on a little personal research project to discover the exact scientific reasons as to why Intermittent Fasting worked so well in my body. I ran into a couple of snags here and there, which have to do with the female only body while fasting. But I went back to the science, read more about what my cells were doing, and then I was able to overcome those snafus to move forward and keep losing weight!

You can keep reading about the scientific evidence that I discovered and wrote about in Chapter 3. You will be as fascinated as I was to discover just exactly what is going on inside you when you either fast or feast. It's pretty eye-opening.

Not to mention life-changing. You won't want to go back to previous ways of dieting or eating, because you will realize that those diets are not in tune with how your body actually works. So, they are doomed to fail! Intermittent Fasting will not doom you to fail. It will launch you towards success.

So, yeah! It's been four years since I've been using Intermittent Fasting to not just lose weight, but to maintain both the healthy weight I am right now and to keep my energy levels nice and high. I have not just high energy levels, but they're stable and do not spike or crash throughout the day.

I discovered many unexpected bonuses that went along with the Intermittent Fasting, too. My weekly meal planning is second nature, plus I have a lot of fun finding and trying new recipes for my eating window times. Grocery shopping is a breeze because I know exactly what foods to buy, and I easily bypass the foods I know will disrupt my current healthy metabolism. I am not a hardcore gym user, but I do get out jogging for about thirty minutes three times a week. That keeps my body healthy and slim. I also train with kettlebells to build up my strength. It helps when carrying things! I sleep better, too. I fall asleep easier, I deeply rest all night long, and I wake up feeling refreshed. My stress levels are down, and I'm able to manage my natural cheerful outlook throughout my life, too. I even feel better during my period, without the sore and heavy chest, sluggish tiredness, brain fog, and irritability I used to experience. Just saying farewell to those symptoms alone is worth it!

I'll talk even more about the benefits of Intermittent Fasting, which you can read all about in Chapter 9 on getting the most out of your diet.

So, are you with me? Would you like to get started on a healthy, doable, totally practical, scientifically based, and enjoyable way to get lean? It's just for women, and it works for women. You'll feel great about the way you look!

What's Included in This Book?

There is a wealth of information in this book that covers all aspects of Intermittent Fasting. You will find all kinds of tips, tricks, dos, don'ts, benefits, troubleshooting tips, and more in here. This is just a sampling of what you will read:

- That One Thing you Need to Know about Intermittent Fasting. It might Change Your Life!
- How Intermittent Fasting stimulates changes in a women's body and how you can use that!
- The different types of Intermittent Fasting and the tips to know which is for you

- Your motivation or motivations to stay on Intermittent Fasting and no its not just willpower!
- The How-To and Not-To when fasting
- Dealing with speed bumps while fasting and how to turn them into Positives!
- What we can learn from a Bear and how this is crucial to weight loss process
- The One Main thing you need to note when comng out of longer fasts
- A complete and detailed 30 day Intermittent Fasting challenge
- What to eat, when to eat, and how to eat during your 30 Day Challenge
- Incorporating the Keto Diet into Intermittent Fasting
- Getting the most out of your Intermittent Fasting journey
- ... and so much more!

There is plenty to learn in this book! You can skip to the chapters that best suit your needs right now, or you can follow my recommendation and read the whole thing straight through from this page to the last. That gives you the most complete picture of Intermittent Fasting, it answer all of your questions in a logical and timely way, and the natural progression of information was laid out here just for you to best understand it. By the time you get to Chapter 8 and the Intermittent Fasting 30 Day Challenge, you'll be inspired to try it. You'll also succeed!

A Fasting Foundation

The next chapter gives you the basics of Intermittent Fasting: its history, what it is, the three types, and the ways you can customize it to fit your lifestyle. Learning these basics gives you the firmest and most solid foundation for succeeding on Intermittent Fasting. As you already know from previous dieting plans in the past, the basics are always more important than they at first appear! Oh, and if you're having trouble with Intermittent Fasting, it also helps to go back to the basics and work on those.

Fast forward towards Intermittent Fasting success!

Chapter 2:
hat is Intermittent Fasting?

Cool, so you want to add Intermittent Fasting to your life and not just shed those pesky pounds, but gain many other rewards along the way!

You definitely can.

In this chapter, we will start with the basics of Intermittent Fasting – what it is, its benefits, its history, and the three types. We'll also examine some of the silly myths around fasting. I want to get you excited to start upon this journey!

So ... What is Intermittent Fasting?

It is exactly what it sounds like!

When you do something intermittently, that means you are not doing it continuously, but in smaller amounts. To fast is to abstain from all foods that have calories for a certain period of time.

When you add those two words together, you get Intermittent Fasting!

This is a scheduled way of combining both extended fasting times and eating times into a continuous routine. It is a way to unlock the exciting features and benefits of Intermittent Fasting, which gives you incredible rewards like:

- A slimmer, trimmer body
- Amazing energy
- Better health
- Having your cells cleaned and revitalized
- Effortless weight loss
- No exercise required!

That is what Intermittent Fasting is designed to do.

But, why has this become a new way of losing weight? What makes it so powerful, and why is it an ideal process for your body to drop the pounds?

Those answers come from how your body actually works and has worked for centuries!

Intermittent Fasting for Human Survival

While in modern times, there is a grocery store or restaurant on every corner ... that was definitely not the case throughout most of human history.

Picture this:

It is thirty thousand years ago, in Europe. It's at the height of summer, but winter is only a few months away. You are expending a lot of calories just doing your daily living. But you're also eating as much as you can while the plants are in season and the animals are plentiful. You eat and eat, basically gorging yourself and eating way more calories than you normally need to survive.

We'll talk more in the next chapter about the science behind food storage in your cells. But thousands of years ago, that's exactly what was happening. Your body stored every tiny extra bit of nutrients in your fat cells. That was their purpose then, and it is still their purpose! You were meant to store extra fuel.

After a few months, the plants died, the animals became scarce, and winter came. Now your body was prepared to face the months and months of vastly reduced food supply. You had spent your summer days storing the food that you needed.

Winter was historically a months' long fasting period. Your body was prepared for it, and your ancestors survived those long, cold winters. You're here!

But your body was built to withstand prolonged fasting times with few calories to sustain you. You were forced to live off of the stored fuel. Consequently, your body switched metabolic states and went into what's called ketosis. Ketosis helped your body use fat as a primary fuel source, not glucose.

Our ancestors survived because their bodies could switch metabolic states so easily, adapt to pretty hardcore fasting, use their stored fuel efficiently, and prevent themselves from starving to death.

Nowadays, though, we live in seriously the most abundant and food plentiful time in human history. Our ancestors would be staggered at the amount of food available to us, the variety, and the constant freshness! They had to make do with whatever they could hunt or gather.

So, that is the history of fasting. It is built into the DNA of each of your cells. Your body was economically designed to conserve and store as much food as humanly possible. It is very efficient and has helped the human race persist and thrive as much as we have for thousands of years.

However, it certainly does not help modern humans like you and me who want to lose that conserved and stored energy! We want to shed that stored fuel, and we want to do it quickly.

The best way to do that?

Turn back the clock on your body. We are going to pretend like it is thirty thousand years ago. We want your body to go into a prolonged fasting mode, so that your existing stored fuel is used. The less stored fuel on your body, the less you weigh. Intermittent Fasting will help you meet those weight loss goals.

That's really all there is to it!

Your Two Fasting Goals

You have two basic goals with Intermittent Fasting:

1. Burn even more fat than you would if you weren't fasting
2. Boost your energy levels

These are not just goals; they're also benefits! In Chapter 3, you will read more about the specific fat burning benefits, and why fasting kicks your metabolism into high gear. You will also read about the science behind why you get so much energy, too.

When we proceed to the preparations before the 30 Day Challenge, you'll be thinking about the weight loss goals to set. It's great to set a small amount of weight to lose, but don't be surprised if your weight loss far surpasses that! Intermittent Fasting is specifically designed to burn fat. Many women have reported astonishing results. You will, too!

Imagine what you would be able to do if you did have plenty of extra energy. Right now, you're probably feeling sluggish from blood spike and crash cycles. Not to mention that your life is pretty busy. You have a full to-do list each day. How can you expect to get it all done?

That is when the power of Intermittent Fasting comes into play. This is an extremely energy boosting way of eating. It lifts up your energy levels to new heights, and helps you accomplish everything you need to do each day – and then some! Wouldn't it be great to feel younger, refreshed, vitalized, and having a natural positive outlook each day? Well, when you decide to both fast the correct way and eat the correct way on Intermittent Fasting schedules, that's really when great stuff happens.

Are You Fasting or Feeding?

Intermittent Fasting is not just about abstaining from food. You are actually going to both eat and not eat on a continuous looping cycle. There are two parts to this cycle:

1. Fasting times

2. Feeding times (also known as eating windows)

You are either in one or the other.

You actually already implement a fasting cycle every day of your life! Did you know that? It's when you are sleeping in between dinner and breakfast. The word "breakfast" literally comes from the phrase "break a fast." Yes, sleeping definitely counts as fasting.

Most of us follow a pretty regular weekly feeding schedule of eating breakfast in the morning, lunch around noon, and dinner in the evening. You fast at night when you sleep. You feed and fast, feed and fast, continuously throughout the weeks and months.

With Intermittent Fasting, we are going to take that same schedule, but just apply more rigidity and structure to it. So, instead of being free to eat whenever you want while you're awake, now you'll have a set period of time when you are supposed to be eating. Also, instead of just fasting when you're asleep, you will also set aside certain hours during the day to fast while you are awake.

Creating your own feeding schedule means that you will set up what are called eating windows. You will be consuming all of that day's calories within the window of time.

Your Intermittent Fasting schedule is now entirely dependent on the clock! Are you feeding or fasting? Depending on the time of day and your Intermittent Fasting schedule, you will know.

The 3 Types of Intermittent Fasting

There are three main types of Intermittent Fasting schedules. Let's take a look at them from easiest to the most challenging.

1. Skipping Meals

You have probably skipped breakfast many times before, especially if you were trying to get to class or work on time.

You just did not know you were Intermittently Fasting at the same time. Skipping meals to extend a fast is definitely the easiest way to continue the benefits of fasting. You could either skip breakfast to extend your fast from the night before, or you could skip dinner to start your nightly fasting time earlier. When you skip meals, you reduce your eating window. You want to make sure you're hitting your calorie count goals before your next fast starts.

2. Fast a Lot, Eat a Little

This is the second most common type of Intermittent Fasting. You stick to a schedule that includes a long period of time fasting followed by a shorter eating window. These eating windows average between six and eight hours per day. Then, you spend the rest of the time fasting. The most common types of this fasting schedule include:

- 8 hour eating window / 16 hour fasting
- 7 hour eating window / 17 hour fasting
- 6 hour eating window / 18 hour fasting

I'll talk a lot more about this version of Intermittent Fasting, because it is the most common and also helps produce amazing results!

3. Multi-Day Fasting

Once you get the hang of Intermittent Fasting and really want to take it to the next level, then you can try fasting for between 24 and up to 36 hours. This is a more complicated, complex version of fasting. You will need to prepare for it, and you will also need to have special mineral rich foods to eat once you come out of the fast, too. In the 30 Day Challenge, I have included two 24-hour long fasts. Those who do the multi-day fasting are especially pleased with the results. I highly recommend becoming proficient enough at fasting that you are able to go for longer periods of time. Don't worry – I'll walk you through all the tips and tricks you need to do it.

In this book I will go into much greater detail about these three types of fasting, how to do them properly, and exactly how to incorporate them into your lifestyle. For now, just be aware of them and start thinking about which type would best fit your schedule. If you are too busy these days with work, family, and other obligations, you might want to just skip meals. For other women, a shorter eating window of six or seven hours is totally doable.

There is no 'right' or 'wrong' way to do Intermittent Fasting. This is a highly customizable form of losing weight. It is custom tailored to you!

Is Fasting Harmful?

Well, since you fast every single night of your life, fasting is definitely not harmful! It is not unhealthy, either. In fact, fasting is a perfectly normal and natural process that gives your body time to rest in between your eating windows.

What about starvation mode? That is when your brain and vital organs start shutting down because they are completely deprived of any food source. No glucose is being consumed and no glucose is stored, either.

Starvation is serious, but Intermittent Fasting never gets that drastic. We are not suggesting you abstain from food for longer than five days at a time! All we are doing is fasting for up to about 36 hours at a time. Those short fasting windows don't produce any starvation adverse effects. Your liver will be using the stored fat in your cells as the ketones for fuel, in place of glucose.

Another misconception about fasting is that it shrinks or depletes your muscle tissue. Yes, it is true that some stored glucose and fat are deposited in some of your muscle cells. But during the fasting times, your body will use those stored fatty acids and not touch your muscle tissue at all! Only during extreme starvation does that happen.

In essence, the short time periods of Intermittent Fasting prevent many of the really bad problems associated with severe fasting and starvation.

So, not to worry! Fasting for up to three days is not harmful. It's all about using up your stored fat and melting that weight right off!

This Will Work for You

Yes, Intermittent Fasting really will work for you. You have the same DNA and the same cells in your body that your ancestors did, and they will act the same way when you fast intermittently!

So, what are you waiting for? Now that you've gotten the basics of fasting, let's go deep into your cells and see what exactly is going on when you're fasting.

Chapter 3:
The Science Behind Intermittent Fasting

I'm pretty geeky, because I love reading about the science behind nutrition. But that's because these are facts! I'd rather have the scientific evidence behind why I do something. I want it to work, and I want it backed up by real claims! It's easy for yet another diet guru to come down the pike and start spouting all kinds of ideas about this diet or that diet.

I prefer to bypass the nonsense and go right to the science.

And, do you know what the science behind Intermittent Fasting and weight loss tells me?

That your body is a fuel-processing machine. It really is! Every single process that goes on in your digestive system is all about receiving fuel, extracting the nutrients, separating those nutrients, getting the right nutrients to the right organs, and then eliminating the waste.

In this chapter, we will talk all about glucose, which is your body's primary fuel source!

Fueling for Fasts

The top three nutrients that you eat in your foods each day:

- Glucose from carbohydrates and sugary foods
- Proteins and amino acids from protein foods like meat and dairy
- Fatty acids from the good fats like olive oil

Glucose is probably the most important sugar of all, because it is such an important energy source. It's also the simplest sugar, being just a monosaccharide. Glucose is made by plants when they photosynthesize, so that's its primary source in your diet. Glucose is absolutely key when it comes to your normal body functioning. It is transformed into glycogen in your body.

We measure this fuel as calories, not glucose consumption – even though that is exactly what's going on. Glucose also comes from several other types of sugars.

When we talk about carbs, we're talking about the three distinct atoms of carbon, hydrogen, and oxygen. The word "carbohydrate" contains these three words. "Carbo" for "carbon," "hydr" for "hydrogen," and "ate" for "oxygen." By themselves, these are three very harmless elements and are the building blocks of life.

But when combined into carbohydrate molecules, these three atoms become a group of sugars, starches, and cellulose (plant sugars) called saccharides. Your body can process four chemical groups of saccharides: the monosaccharides, disaccharides, oligosaccharides, and polysaccharides. It is the fourth group, the polysaccharides, that are processed by the body and then stored as energy in your cells.

Sugars are even less complex carbohydrates than the saccharides. They come in many other forms besides glucose, including:

Sucrose (table sugar)

This is the regular sweet white or brown sugar you can purchase in stores that's also found in so many food items, especially baked goods. Table sugar comes from the stems of the sugarcane plant and the roots of the sugar beet. It also contains cellulose plant sugars.

Fructose (fruit sugar)

This is what gives fruits like strawberries, cherries, bananas, and apples their characteristic sweetness. It is also present in some natural sweeteners like honey and agave. Fructose is a monosaccharide sugar. It can also bond to glucose and form sucrose. Fructose is easily made into syrups, like the high fructose corn syrup that's so prevalent in foods these days.

Cellulose (plant sugar)

Cellulose is a polysaccharide sugar that's found in plant cell walls and certain vegetable fibers. Some of your favorite vegetables have really high amounts of cellulose. That includes potatoes, carrots, and corn. Humans can't digest cellulose, so it's usually broken down into its smaller glucose molecules and – you guessed it – stored in your cells for future energy.

Lactose (milk sugar)

People who are lactose intolerant can't digest milk sugars, which are disaccharides made up of galactose and glucose. Cows' milk is really high in lactose. Dairy cheeses have smaller amounts of lactose.

Too Much Fuel = Stored Fat

"Fat" is just a short term nickname for the fatty acids that are present in fats. Fatty acids are long chains of molecules with different chemical components that are various combinations of three atoms: carbon, hydrogen, and oxygen.

Too much of a good thing really is too much, in this case.

Did you know that all three types of fuel – glycogen, proteins, and fatty acids – can be stored as excess in your cells?

Which cells are they stored in? Those cells are called adipocyte cells, which are made of adipose tissue. That adipose tissue's entire specialty in life is to store that excess fuel or excess energy. Think of adipocyte cells as little tiny storage centers all over your body.

Carbohydrates provide fuel, contribute towards stabilizing your blood sugar, and are also frequently found in many fibrous foods like seeds, nuts, legumes, and vegetables.

It is when you eat too many carbohydrates, but especially glucose (which is found in regular sugar, fructose and cellulose), that things start to go haywire. Your health will start to take a turn for the worst, and you'll also notice the weight gain, too.

After you eat good fats, your cells break them down into both glycerol and those fatty acids. This process is called lipolysis. Both the glycerol and those fatty acids are released into your blood and travel through your bloodstream to your liver.

That's where those same fatty acids can then be either broken down directly and used for that day's energy, or they can enter into a new multiple step process called gluconeogenesis, which turns those fatty acids into glucose. Amino acids are combined with the fatty acids to manufacture glucose. Then the glucose is used the same way as other carbohydrates are processed, which is explained below.

What about extra fats? Are those used as energy, like glycogen, or are they stored, like excess protein and carbohydrates?

The answer is yes: those fats are stored. They are stored as triglycerides in fat cells called adipocytes. Those cells can expand, but they do have a limit. In addition, that stored fat can also be stored in your muscles to provide extra energy for when you need it. When you're doing moderate intensity exercising, your muscles open up those stored fat cells and use that energy to meet your fuel needs.

After you eat your protein serving, it is digested in the stomach and absorbed by the intestines. Then it goes directly to your liver, where the nitrogen and the amino acids are broken down and separated. Your amino acids are sent to your muscles for fuel. There are nine essential amino acids in protein, and if all of those are present, then your body uses them all up happily. However, any excess protein that's not used by your body is then turned into either glucose (sugar) or fatty acids and sent to your cells for energy and storage purposes.

That's right. If you eat too much protein, it is stored and causes you to gain weight!

Excess Fuel Storage = Excess Pounds to Lose

Now that you've learned exactly how your body processes each nutrient (carbohydrates, fats, and proteins), let's put the whole scenario together in a real-life example.

This is exactly what's happening in your body every day of your life!

Let's say that you eat a balanced dinner with chicken, potatoes, green peas, and an orange. The chicken is made primarily up of proteins and the good fats. The potatoes are carbohydrates, mostly starches, cellulose (plant sugar), and glucose. Both the green peas and the orange are made up of fructose (fruit sugar), cellulose (plant sugar), and glucose.

Then let's say that after you ate this dinner, you watched a half-hour show on TV, and then took your dog out for a fifteen-minute walk around the block. Well, in that time frame, you are going to use a certain portion of that fuel that you just ate at dinner. You will use the proteins and amino acids and fats from the chicken. You will also use the sugars from the orange, potatoes, and peas, which all have been processed into glycogen.

But you won't use all of that fuel. The rest is stored in that adipose tissue present in your adipocyte cells. There are two storage processes: glycogenesis and lipogenesis.

- Glycogenesis is when excess glucose is converted into glycogen and stored in your liver and muscles. Your body stores up to 2000 calories of this! If you fast for up to 24 hours with no incoming glucose, then your body will use this glycogen storage first.

24

- Lipogenesis is when there's enough glycogen in your muscles and liver, so the glucose is converted into fat and stored in those adipocyte cells. Your fat stores are pretty unlimited, unfortunately. This is the kind of storage we're trying to shed!

That extra fuel is stored for as long as it needs to be, until your body requires it during a time of calorie and nutritional deficiency. Historically, this would have been winter! Today though, our modern American culture doesn't have a starvation period.

Still, your body just keeps on storing those excess nutrients. Too much fuel of all three kinds (proteins, fats, and carbohydrates) makes you gain weight.

That is the real picture of what's going on inside your body.

You ate plenty of the right types of fuel. It was just too much of it!

So, now you want to shed your extra fuel storage. It would be so much easier if we could just reach inside those adipocyte cells and extract that storage. That process would be similar to decluttering your basement. You want to get rid of the excess fuel storage that you've been carrying around for months or even years.

Intermittent Fasting is the most natural way to declutter all of this extra fuel storage that you want to shed from your body.

Fasting Burns Fuel Storage

While we can't just mentally tell our adipocyte cells to start decluttering, Intermittent Fasting is the process that kickstarts your body into doing that!

On a typical day, you eat a lot of those three types of fuel sources – carbohydrates, fats, and proteins. That's plenty of incoming glucose to store as glycogen or convert to fat and store.

But what if you stop eating and start fasting instead? When your body isn't receiving any more incoming fuel sources, what does it do then?

Well, you still need energy to run your brain, organs, skeleton, and muscles. You still need fuel. So, your cells look elsewhere for that fuel source. That's why they go right to those adipocyte cells, into the adipose tissue, and start extracting the stored fuel.

The whole process looks like this:

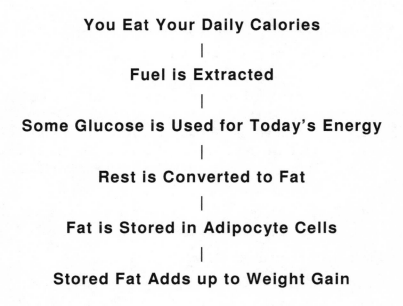

You Eat Your Daily Calories

|

Fuel is Extracted

|

Some Glucose is Used for Today's Energy

|

Rest is Converted to Fat

|

Fat is Stored in Adipocyte Cells

|

Stored Fat Adds up to Weight Gain

This is what's currently happening, and the whole process happens every day inside your body. It's very gradual, but it adds up to increased weight gain over time.

Unfortunately, the absolutely domineering message in our American food culture is that we are eating the wrong things! Too much fat, too many carbohydrates, too little protein, and on and on it goes.

But, as you've seen in this chapter, it's not so much that we are eating the wrong types of fuel. Your body is extremely well adapted to process carbohydrates, fats, and proteins.

It's that we're eating too much and too often!

The more you eat, the more excess glucose is converted to fat and stored in your adipocyte cells.

It really comes down to this:

Eat Larger, Healthier Meals Less Often

That's a very good mantra to post on your wall, on your fridge, or in your kitchen somewhere. It will help you stay focused on the bigger picture!

You're going to eat larger meals less often than you have been eating your regular three meals a day plus snacks, and you're going to eat healthier ingredients. We will definitely cover which ingredients in the next chapter!

Then on top of this mantra, we're going to add Intermittent Fasting periods to your weekly schedule.

Putting All the Pieces Together

What does your body do after you've eaten all your meals for the day? I'm glad you asked!

After your eating window is done and you're fasting, your body has to seek elsewhere for fuel.

Here is what that process looks like:

You Stop Eating and Fast for 18 Hours

|

No Additional Glucose or Proteins or Fatty Acids Enter the Body

|

Cells Still Need Fuel

|

Cells Extract Stored Fat from Adipocyte Cells

|

Fat is Sent to Liver for Processing

|

Liver Turns Fat into Ketones (called Ketogenesis)

Ketones Used as Fuel

The more consistently you keep up a fasting schedule, the more weight that you lose! That is because your liver is using all that stored fat to make ketones.

What are ketones? Ketones are small organic compounds of fuel made up of carbon and oxygen that are bonded to hydrocarbon groups. That's a fancy scientific way of saying they are an alternate fuel source to fatty acids, proteins, and the glucose from carbohydrates.

When your body is subsisting primarily on ketones for fuel rather than glucose, you are said to be in ketosis. We'll talk more about that in Chapter 10 when discussing the Keto Diet. Many of you will want to get into ketosis and stay there, because you are consistently burning more of that stored fat in your adipocyte cells.

But, you don't have to be on a special diet for your body to use stored fuel. You're just going to eat larger, healthier meals less often.

The Intermittent Fasting will help you take care of the rest!

How Intermittent Fasting Affects Women

So now, you know exactly how your body processes carbohydrates to turn them into glucose and glycogen, fats to turn them into fatty acids, and proteins to turn them into proteins and amino acids.

Yet, there are so many other ways that Intermittent Fasting affects your body. We are not just different than men physically. We are also affected differently when we abstain from eating. Since so much of the female body and our monthly cycle is about preparing for pregnancy and carrying healthy babies, getting the proper nutrients is of the utmost importance. That is why fasting from foods is such a big deal for women. In some ways, we don't have all of the positive benefits that men experience.

So, when you fast, there are certain side effects that you will definitely notice. Let's go through them one by one to explain what they are and what you should expect when you fast.

Your Ovulation Hormones

Intermittent Fasting definitely affects your hormones. Your body is so sensitive to calorie restriction. So, when your calorie intake is low, from fasting for long periods of time, that affects the hypothalamus in your brain. This in turn disrupts the secretion of a hormone called gonadotropin (GnRH). GnRH helps release two reproductive hormones, luteinizing hormone (LH) and follicle stimulating hormone (FSH).

Those two reproductive hormones – LH and FSH – are the ones that communicate with your ovaries to release eggs each month. They trigger the production of both estrogen and progesterone, which are needed to release an egg each month so you can either become pregnant or have your period in your normal 28-day cycle.

But, when those hormones aren't released and there is no communication with your ovaries, that definitely affects your ovulation cycle. No egg is released, because the hormones haven't told it to. Your periods might become irregular, and it can cause problems with fertility, too. This is especially true if you spend a long time on Intermittent Fasting, going up to three to six months at a time or longer. It even causes a reduction in ovary size and irregular reproductive cycles. Some women have reported, and this is in more extreme cases, that it brings on early-onset menopause.

From a historical standpoint, this makes sense! Thousands of years ago when times of food were scarce, the last thing your body wanted to do was bring a baby into the world. It was too high a risk for the infant and the mother, who would probably starve. Your body doesn't know it's the 21st century. So, Intermittent Fasting definitely affects your ovulation cycle.

Your Hunger Hormones

Fasting also affects three hormones that both regulate and react to either hunger or satiety – leptin, insulin, and ghrelin. These hormones' goals are to maintain homeostasis, which keeps everything in balance. That means not too much hunger or too little, as well as not feeling too full or not enough. When you fast and reduce the calories you eat compared to what you're burning, you get hungry.

Both leptin and ghrelin regulate appetite. Leptin is secreted primarily from your fat cells, but also in your stomach – it decreases hunger. Whereas ghrelin is secreted in your stomach lining, and it increases hunger. Both of them are responding to how much you eat!

When you fast, you're reducing those fat cells and secreting a lot of leptin! It decreases your hunger, making you feel less inclined to eat those calories. Oh, cool! You're thinking. I can just fast and won't feel hungry? That's awesome! Well, not so fast. You still have to take in enough calories to eat during the day. We'll talk more about that in the next chapter.

As for ghrelin, that's the 'rumbling in your stomach' hormone, causing you to go to the fridge or poking through cupboards. When your stomach is empty, it makes ghrelin, which travels through your blood up to your brain and triggers that peckish feeling. When studies have been done on ghrelin, scientists have been surprised to discover the levels have stayed stable during longer fasts up to 33 hours. So, eating nothing for a day makes you no more or less hungry! As a bonus, being a woman, your ghrelin hunger hormone decreases much, much faster than a man's when you abstain from eating. So, you will feel less and less hungry the longer you fast.

Your Thyroid

How does Intermittent Fasting affect your thyroid? For women with thyroid conditions, like hypothyroidism, can Intermittent Fasting help you with thyroid issues? Fasting decreases the concentration of the T3 thyroid hormone, while the T4 (thyroxine) levels stay the same. The thyroid stimulating hormone TSH does not increase, either. These changes only occur if you do more serious multi-day fasting, like three days or longer.

So, in effect, when you fast for two days or just Intermittently each day, that has very little scientific bearing on your thyroid function. You're free to continue managing your thyroid condition the same as you would if you weren't fasting.

Your Sleeping Patterns

Another side effect of Intermittent Fasting is that your normal sleeping patterns get disrupted. You'll find you have difficulty getting to sleep, staying asleep, and waking up feeling refreshed. This is especially the case if your shorter eating window is a big change from any previous meal time habits. While this is unfortunate and makes you feel tired, it actually clears up after about a week or so. That's because your circadian rhythm needs some time to adapt, just like when you deal with jet lag by crossing time zones.

Like the hormones, this also has to do with brain function. Your brain needs hours of sleep in order to perform all its processes when you wake back up, like reading, learning, memorizing, coming up with new ideas, remembering, thinking, and everything else. After you get used to Intermittent Fasting, you'll find that it helps to make you feel more calm and grounded throughout the day, with less nervousness, tension, anxiety, and stress.

Remember that your body adapts very well to Intermittent Fasting because this was such a necessary survival mechanism centuries ago.

None of these side effects are guaranteed for every woman who tries Intermittent Fasting! But if you do have them, now you know why. You're advised to keep your fasting to a minimum of every two or three days.

Some women pick up fasting with no problem, have no issue with it, and don't experience any of these symptoms at all. Everybody is different.

Positive Body Changes!

When you incorporate Intermittent Fasting into your life, you are going to see some wonderful and positive body changes!

As you've read in this chapter, there is an amazing wealth of scientific information out there as to how your body processes every nutrient you eat. So, exactly what kinds of foods are you going to be eating in between your times fasting?

I'm so glad you asked, since I love to talk about food. Who doesn't, right? That is exactly what we'll discuss in the next chapter.

Chapter 4:
Eating as Part of Intermittent Fasting

As you can see, Intermittent Fasting has so much to do with what you're eating during the day! In this chapter, I want to talk about what exactly you will be eating, your calories, and ways to make eating fun on this diet.

We came up with an amazing mantra in the last chapter about how to eat in between your fasting times.

Eat Larger, Healthier Meals Less Often

Yep, we're going to kick a lot of eating myths right to the curb. Myths about three meals a day, myths about small portion sizes, myths about eating the wrong things, myths about eating the right things, and myths about calories or calorie counting.

Intermittent Fasting is about four huge eating concepts:

1. Eating in a small, specific window of time, within 8 hours or less
2. Eating healthy meals that contain proteins, carbohydrates, and fats
3. Eating fewer meals, usually two or even one a day instead of three a day plus snacks
4. Eating to meet your calorie requirements

We'll go over each one of these in-depth in this chapter, starting with calories!

Calories and Intermittent Fasting

Calories were discovered by Nicolas Clement in 1824 as a unit of heat energy. But nowadays, we think of calories as the basic unit of how food will burn as fuel in your body.

What is your recommended daily calorie intake? In other words, how many calories does your particular body require to maintain that balance your own body is looking for?

To find out how many calories you need to eat, just go to an online calorie calculator. You will fill in your information, including your age, your current weight, and your height. You will also provide your current level of weekly exercise. This is to determine whether you're burning more calories than you currently take in.

You know calories because they're listed on food packages or you can Google them, right? Most of us who've been dieting for some time actually have a pretty firm grasp of how many calories are in fruits, vegetables, meats, dairy, and grains. No biggie there.

For women, the average amount of calories is about 1800 per day. That depends on many factors, but it is a nice round number and a good place to start. That's your base level.

Did you know that you can actually eat more calories and lose more weight just by adding Intermittent Fasting?

Whoa! That's pretty life changing.

Let's take an average 1800 calorie day. You split up your calories throughout the day, eating several hundred for breakfast, several hundred for lunch, some for an afternoon snack, several hundred for dinner, and the rest in the evening. Even though you're proud of yourself for getting in a lower calorie diet, you're running into several problems:

- Lower calorie foods just don't fill you up and satisfy your hunger, so you feel pretty ravenous throughout the day.
- You're not eating a lot of calories, but you are eating frequently.

You're not eating too many calories, but you are eating too often!

On the Intermittent Fasting eating plan, you can eat up to 2000 calories per day in a shorter eating window – and lose weight faster!

Yes, it's absolutely true.

How is that even possible?

It's because of how your body processes the nutrients from your foods. We talked a lot about nutrients back in Chapter 3, and the three main nutrients are fats, proteins, and carbohydrates.

Your body actually prefers if you consume lots of these nutrients in one sitting. We're talking 1000 calories in one meal. In our modern era, it's almost unheard of to try and eat so much in one meal unless you're trying to gain weight. But you split up all of those 2000 calories into just two meals a day, at 1000 calories each, and get rid of all snacking in between. You eat those two meals within a 6-hour window. Then, you fast the rest of the time. You'd actually feel incredibly full longer, you'd meet all of your calorie requirements, and you'd lose more weight because you ate enough fuel and nutrients to not just sustain yourself during the fast, but increase the rate at which that fat from your adipose cells are burned.

Pretty incredible, huh?

It's still a good idea to get your base calories for your body type and fitness level, just to give yourself a baseline number. But you can safely stick to a 2000 calorie diet on the Intermittent Fasting plan – and still drop those pounds.

Losing weight is NOT just about cutting calories! That is the standard conventional wisdom, but we have much more scientific evidence to back up our claims and provide you with all the information you need.

Cutting calories is also NOT the only possible way to lose weight. If that were true, then every single person who ever ate fewer calories would automatically start dropping the pounds. That would be a magical weight loss fantasy indeed! But that's not what is happening.

Thankfully, more and more women are waking up to the fact that simply cutting your calories doesn't work for weight loss. This is one of the many reasons why Intermittent Fasting and the Keto Diet have suddenly jumped in popularity.

You are free to eat up to 2000 calories a day, and still lose weight.

Hallelujah!

Okay, So What Should I Be Eating?

Well, just because you can eat 2000 calories per day doesn't mean those calories should come from junk. We want to eat healthy! Intermittent Fasting is all about eating windows, which I'll talk about below. But before we get there, let's talk about exactly what kinds of foods you should be eating. Remember that you can eat up to 2000 calories, so we're not dealing with restrictive diets.

We're dealing with healthy, balanced diets. Diets that contain healthy amounts of those three awesome nutrients we were talking about earlier:

- Carbohydrates (starches and sugars)
- Proteins

- Fats

So, a healthy diet would include healthy amounts of each of those three nutrients. While you have a lot of leeway here, the percentages that I have personally used in the past are:

- Carbohydrates – 40% of daily total calories
- Proteins – 30% of daily total calories
- Fats – 30% of daily total fats

This means that on a 2000 calorie diet, you'd be eating 800 calories of healthy carbohydrates, 600 calories of healthy proteins, and 600 calories of healthy fats each day.

You have a lot of flexibility here – an entire grocery store's worth, actually!

There are a number of diets out there to choose from, like Atkins, the Paleo Diet, or the Ketogenic Diet, which is discussed in depth in Chapter 10. You could even go vegetarian or vegan if you like! Again, Intermittent Fasting is more about when you're eating your calories, not so much exactly what those calories should be.

However, common sense tells us that calories from fried foods aren't the same as calories from organic chicken. Eating 2000 calories in larger meals is not a carte blanche excuse to just go crazy. Healthy is key. There are good and bad carbohydrates, good and bad proteins, and good and bad fats. You want to stay away from the bad kinds and choose the good kinds.

Speaking of grocery stores, let's go shopping and take a look at each of the food groups to see which foods fall under the healthy category.

<u>Vegetables</u>

The produce section has some wonderful options to get in your healthy carbohydrates. You can't go wrong with leafy greens like Romaine lettuce, fresh baby spinach, and kale. They make a great base to salads. You can also eat onions, tomatoes (although they're a fruit), broccoli, cabbage, cauliflower, celery, cucumbers, green peas, fresh green beans, bell peppers, beets, Brussel sprouts, carrots, squash, zucchini, eggplant, and asparagus. Starchier veggies like potatoes, sweet potatoes / yams, and turnips have higher carbohydrate counts if you're watching those numbers.

Fruits

Many diets, especially the Keto Diet, advocate a very low carbohydrate gram count that doesn't include hardly any fruits. But fruits are high carbohydrate foods with lots of natural fructose, which can convert to glucose and provide great energy for your body. Excellent healthy fruits include apples, oranges, bananas, berries, grapes, pineapple, lemons, limes, and melons. Avocados are popular, too.

Eggs & Dairy

Dairy foods provide proteins, some lactose (milk sugar), and good fats, too. Try to get dairy products either organic or grass-fed, since those are the healthiest and provide you with the best protein sources. Milk, cream, real butter, cottage cheese, cream cheese, plain unsweetened yogurt, goat cheese, and other types of cheeses will give you yummy calories. Whole large eggs are a versatile food that also have plenty of good fats and proteins.

Meat & Fish

It's perfectly fine to get all of your calories from non-meat sources on a vegetarian diet with Intermittent Fasting. But you can also get your proteins from sources like chicken, turkey, beef, ham, high quality bacon, lamb, fish, and seafood like clams, shrimp, scallops, crab, and lobster. Buy good quality meat and fish. They'll provide plenty of proteins and the good kinds of fats to meet your calorie requirements.

Carbs & Grains

The carbohydrate category is one of the more controversial, because those carbohydrates from flours, sugars, and starches convert right to glucose in your body. On the Keto Diet, your carbohydrate count is 25 grams or less. But if you're following an Intermittent Fasting plan with more carbs, then you can increase the count. Don't go overboard in this category, though! You want some good fats and proteins, too. Examples of great carbs that have plenty of fiber and give you long-lasting energy include oats, barley, quinoa, lentils, beans (kidney, cannellini, navy, black beans), brown rice, wild rice, chickpeas, and bran. As for breads, you can get whole wheat, rye, pumpernickel, or sprouted grain. Try to keep your corn, white rice, and white flour consumption to a very small percentage of your carbohydrate intake.

Herbs & Spices

Herbs and spices have their own very low carbohydrate counts because of the plant sugars. They add their own unique and amazing flavors to the above food groups. You can change up cuisines and eat different kinds of dishes. You can find fresh herbs and garlic in the produce section, but you should also stock plenty of dried herbs and spices, too. One fun thing about cooking is getting to try a new herb or spice you're not familiar with. Herbs and spices pack a punch with flavor that excites your taste buds and turn healthy ingredients from blah to blasting.

More Healthy Foods

There are hundreds of other healthy ingredients that you can add to your cupboards, fridge, and freezer. You can try the different types of nuts and seeds. There are many healthy condiments like olive oil, balsamic vinegar, soy sauce, Dijon mustard, low sugar barbecue sauce, full fat mayonnaise, and hot sauce. Black coffee and teas can be mixed with cream. Some

Intermittent Fasters stock baking ingredients. It's up to you whether you'd like to have sugars. Remember that they convert to glucose and become stored in your cells.

Treats

Yes, you can have some treats on this diet! Dark chocolate is yummy, and so is a glass of wine. Many ice cream brands are pretty healthy, so look for ones that are just milk, cream, sugar, and natural ingredients. Even pizzas and French fries have healthy versions. Whatever your personal indulgence is, keep note of it. You don't have to write it off completely. Just have a tiny portion of it with as few artificial ingredients as possible, factor in the calories, and only have it occasionally, like once a week. This is not a meal plan about deprivation.

Any Off-Limit Foods?

While it's more important when you eat in between your fasting times, there are certain foods you shouldn't be eating on this diet. That is because they're just plain unhealthy! They are made in a laboratory, so that makes them stuffed with artificial sweeteners, colors, flavors, and preservatives. These chemicals are the bad kinds of carbohydrates, fats, and proteins. They're not all natural straight from the ground or the animal.

Avoid:

- Boxed pastries and baked goods
- Margarine in any form
- Canned soups
- Canned meals (Chef Boyardee, etc.)
- Boxed meal kits
- Frozen boxed lunches or dinners
- Frozen breakfast foods
- Frozen pizza
- Kids' lunch packaged meals

- Grocery store packaged foods
- Pre-packaged sauce mixes
- Dried soup mixes
- Potato chips
- Cheesy crunchy snacks
- Bagged microwave popcorn
- Cheese crackers
- Any packaged salty or cheese snack food
- High sugar coffee drinks from Starbucks or other coffee shops
- Soda, even if it says zero calories
- Energy drinks
- Sports drinks
- Alcohol, unless it's the occasional glass of wine

Most of these are pretty self-explanatory as to why they are on the naughty list. They're packed with nasty ingredients like high fructose corn syrup, trans fats, and manufactured items like partially hydrogenated oil, aspartame, xylitol, and dextrose. Not to mention the ridiculously high amounts of sodium, caffeine, and sugars.

Yuck!

Honestly, anything packed with seventy ingredients you can't pronounce is not good for your wonderful body. Stick to an eating plan that works for you, incorporates at least 90% good, healthy ingredients, and provides you with those amazing carbs, proteins, and good fats.

Your Eating Windows

The Intermittent Fasting plan focuses more on WHEN you eat! We're going to squeeze all of your 2000 calories into a shorter period of time than the average day. Most of us begin eating in the morning, and we don't pay attention to the clock. We might have our last bite or two very late at night.

That's not going to work with Intermittent Fasting. Your diet is not just dependent upon what you put in the grocery cart.

It's about the clock, too.

So, the maximum amount of time you should be eating for weight loss is a 9 hour daily window. A minimum time is about 5 hours, but that's only if you are doing one meal a day (OMAD), which I will discuss in more detail below.

You get a lot of flexibility with choosing how long your eating window is.

Eating Window Examples:

- Eating window of 9 hours, fast for 15 hours, repeat
- Eating window of 8 hours, fast for 16 hours, repeat
- Eating window of 7 hours, fast for 17 hours, repeat
- Eating window of 6 hours, fast for 18 hours, repeat
- Eating window of 5 hours, fast for 19 hours, repeat

You can see that your eating windows and fasting times keep repeating, over and over, on that cycle.

Which one is best for you? I personally have found the shorter eating windows of 6 or 7 hours to be the most effective for weight loss. I am just not hungry in the morning, so my eating window starts at noon and stops at 7:00 pm each day. I eat all of my 2000 calories within that time frame. I eat 30% of my calories at lunch at 12:00 pm noon, and then have a 70% calorie dinner at 5:30 pm. I like to eat a lot at dinner! Once that clock hits 7:00 pm, I stop for the day.

That is how an eating window works.

The 8 Hour Eating Window and the Hunger Hormone

Remember back in Chapter 3 I mentioned the hunger hormone, called ghrelin?

Well, it turns out this hunger hormone lives on its own natural 8 hour eating window every single day of your life.

Ghrelin levels are pretty low even after you wake up, those levels peak at noon, and then those levels steadily decrease throughout the day, corresponding with a smaller peak around 8:00 pm at night. Sound familiar? You are definitely your hungriest at lunch time, throughout the afternoon, and at dinner. Millions of people skip breakfast not necessarily because we're trying to, but because those ghrelin levels are low. We're simply not hungry!

These ghrelin levels also give you the most perfect 8 hour eating window between 12:00 pm and 8:00 pm. Pretty neat, huh? It's like you were biologically designed to have this 8 hour eating window. Your ghrelin hunger hormone levels certainly support it. This is an eating window that works with your body, rather than against it.

The only rule of thumb when it comes to finding the best eating window of time, is that your last meal should occur about two to three hours before bedtime. Eating windows of time last around six hours, which gives you eighteen hours of fasting. So, for example, if you go to bed at 11:00 at night, your six-hour feeding window could be between 3:00 pm and 9:00 pm. That's the latest it could be. This is a perfectly fine Intermittent Fasting eating schedule.

Here are some possible examples:

- Have a full time nine to five job? Try an eating window between 7:00 am and 1:00 pm. Take in most of your calories at breakfast and then the rest at a noon lunch time.
- Work a late shift? Schedule your feeding window between 9:00 am and 3:00 pm, in the middle of the day before your shift starts.

- An early riser? Then your eating window can be between 5:00 am and 11:00 am. You'd take in all of your calories in the morning.
- What about the night owl? Your eating window is shifted to later in the day, starting at 3:00 pm and ending at 11:00 pm. If you have a very late bed time of 1:00 in the morning, this would be a great time for you.

Spend some time looking at your weekly schedule to find the best times that work for you.

Splitting Up Your Calories in the Eating Window

The percentages of calories that you're consuming at each of your meals in your eating window is really important. Consistency is key on the Intermittent Fasting plan, so whatever calorie percentage template you use, please keep repeating it for each of your eating windows.

You get several options here of how many meals you'd like to have. I started out with three meals per day within a 9 hour eating window. That was because I wasn't sure if I would be ravenous with having to fast for the other 15 hours. I also was still locked into the mindset of 'three meals a day is normal.' In fact, I was more used to eating six meals a day, because I ate smaller portion sizes and just grazed all day! That is not a meal plan for weight loss – that's a meal plan for weight gain!

So, on the Intermittent Fasting eating plan, you can cut back from three meals a day to just two or even try one meal a day (OMAD).

Sample Templates: 8 Hour Eating Window with Three Meals a Day

This is an excellent beginning sample template for starting out with Intermittent Fasting and getting used to the whole process. It's also perfect for women who are in college taking classes, women who work full time, and women who would

45

like smaller portions rather than eating two larger meals per day. For the times, you can definitely move your eating window to be earlier in the day or later in the day.

Your schedule could look like this:

- Meal 1 is between 12:00 pm and 2:00 pm, when you eat 30% of your calories.
- Meal 2 is between 3:00 pm and 5:00 pm and that is when you eat another 30% of your calories.
- Meal 3 is between 6:00 pm and finishes before 8:00 pm, when you consume 40% of your calories.

This template is really balanced.

You could still follow this template with the exact same number of meals, but only the calorie percentages are switched.

- Meal 1 is between 12:00 pm and 2:00 pm, when you eat 30% of your calories.
- Meal 2 is between 3:00 pm and 5:00 pm and that is when you eat another 20% of your calories.
- Meal 3 is between 6:00 pm and finishes before 8:00 pm, when you consume 50% of your calories.

For busy moms with families when dinner is the biggest meal of the day, this template would be ideal. You would have a large dinner with your family in the evening.

Do you work a later shift or have more time earlier in the day to get in most of your calories? If you are a breakfast lover within your 8 hour eating window, then check out the following meal plan template:

- Meal 1 is between 6:00 am and 8:00 am, when you eat 60% of your calories.
- Meal 2 is between 10:00 am and 11:00 am and that is when you eat another 15% of your calories.

- Meal 3 is between 12:00 pm and finishes before 2:00 pm, when you consume 25% of your calories.

Notice that I also moved the eating window up to starting at 6:00 am instead of 12:00 pm? That is the power of eating windows. You can start them at any time you want. The important thing is to stop all food consumption at the end of the eating window and fast until the eating window starts again tomorrow. You can have water, but that's it. No other calories!

All of these meal percentages were for 8 hours. You can certainly shorten the time frame down to 7 hours and use the same percentages.

Sample Templates: 8 Hour Eating Window with Two Meals a Day

Now that you've gotten an idea of what exactly Intermittent Fasting looks like on a three meal a day plan, we are going to stick with the same eating window time of 8 hours. But this time, we will reduce your meals from three to two. This also changes the calorie ercentage. You will consume more calories per sitting. Many of us skip breakfast, so eating just two meals a day comes naturally! I've eaten two meals a day for years, and I feel so much fuller and so much better. Think back to 30,000 years ago. Our ancestors could probably only eat once or twice a day, because the rest of the time was needed for actually hunting the food! It is very natural to eat just two meals a day.

For an 8 hour eating window, your schedule could look like this:

- Meal 1 is between 12:00 pm and 2:00 pm, when you eat 30% of your calories.
- Meal 2 is between 6:00 pm and finishes before 8:00 pm, when you consume 70% of your calories.

I call this the Dinner Lover template! If you love to have a sit down supper with your family in the evening, then you would try this template. Keep in mind that a two meal a day plan does not provide any calories for snacking in between meals. You are consuming all of your calories within two meals, and in two meals only.

What about if you need to or want to eat the vast majority of your calories earlier in the day? You could definitely do that in your 8 hour eating window.

- Meal 1 is between 12:00 pm and 2:00 pm, when you eat 70% of your calories.
- Meal 2 is between 6:00 pm and finishes before 8:00 pm, when you consume 30% of your calories.

Don't forget that you could move your eating window earlier, to consume that 70% of your calories starting at six in the morning if that fits in your schedule. If you do that, you would plan your second meal so that it stops at 2:00 pm.

Sample Template: 6 Hour Eating Window with Two Meals a Day

The longer you fast, the more weight you will lose. So, many women love to increase their fasting times, shortening their eating windows to 6 hours instead of the usual 8. You will gain more and more benefits from fasting from longer periods of time. In a 6 hour eating window, you really only have enough time to enjoy two large meals. You can split up the calorie percentages to have it be either top heavy (most of your calories in the beginning) or bottom heavy (most of your calories at the end).

Check out this sample 6 hour eating window with two meals:

- Meal 1 is between 12:00 pm and 2:00 pm, when you eat 70% of your calories.

- Meal 2 is between 4:00 pm and finishes before 6:00 pm, when you consume 30% of your calories.

This is the top heavy version, where you have a huge lunch. Would you rather have a huge dinner? That is great, too! You could reverse the calorie percentage for your 6 hours:

- Meal 1 is between 12:00 pm and 2:00 pm, when you eat 30% of your calories.
- Meal 2 is between 4:00 pm and finishes before 6:00 pm, when you consume 70% of your calories.

As with the 8 hour eating windows above, you can move this eating window to be earlier in the day or later in the day. Just make sure that you are finishing your meals before the end of the 6 hour eating window and that you are having your last bite at least two hours before bed time.

One Meal a Day Intermittent Fasting - OMAD

Now, we get to the pinnacle of the amazingness of Intermittent Fasting, and that is consuming just one meal a day (OMAD for short). Yes, that is right – you would eat all 2000 calories in a single sitting. But that also means it is your only meal that day, and you are not to eat any other calories and have no other foods until you break your fast tomorrow to eat your 2000 calories again. So, it is more difficult than simply reducing meals or playing around with calorie percentages like in the above sample template meal plans.

However, there are some awesome perks to eating OMAD:

- You can eat your OMAD whenever you want – have fun picking the time that works best for you
- Forget planning multiple meals – now you can just find about 1 hour each day in which to eat. That's it!
- You only have to cook once a day, for just one huge meal
- You will feel like an Olympic athlete consuming that many calories in a single sitting

- You will greatly simplify your grocery shopping and meal planning
- After you have eaten your OMAD, you don't have to think about food the rest of the day

With OMAD, the ratio is 23:1. So, you are fasting for about twenty-three hours and only eating for one hour. Eating just once a day is extraordinarily beneficial for women who have very busy lives, who travel frequently, who are stay at home moms, who have a full college course load, who are high performance athletes, and for any woman who would love to just eat all their calories in one huge sitting. It's like having your own personal banquet each day!

There are some tips to eating OMAD, because of how your body processes those key nutrients. If you are doing OMAD specifically for weight loss purposes, you would want to try and reduce your carbohydrate count down to about 15% of your daily calories or less. That is because the less glucose you consume, the fewer grams turn into glycogen and the more fat is used as fuel from your adipose cells. You might also want to try the full Keto Diet, with is extremely low carb counts that kick your body into ketosis much faster and use up that stored fat for ketones. Read about the Keto Diet in Chapter 10.

The other tip to eating OMAD is to ease into it slowly. This is not an eating plan about deprivation. 2000 calories is a lot to consume in one sitting! But the other twenty three hours of fasting is a long time. So, go easy on yourself. You are used to eating multiple meals a day, so there is an issue about changing your mindset, too.

The third tip? Keep that huge meal stuffed full of good, healthy nutrients. When eating just once a day, you could be tempted to just binge on one type of food. But you want to be sure you're getting enough variety. This is not an eating plan that will work if it becomes boring! Change up your flavors with each of your single meals. You will deeply enjoy eating and fall in love with this meal plan.

Difficult fasts don't equal better results if you're feeling deprived. You don't get bonus points for starvation or deprivation. You just feel deprived.

So, find an eating window and a meal plan that works for you!

Eating by the Calendar and the Clock

Your eating window is as unique to your lifestyle as you are! That's because it starts with your weekly calendar and how you can find the best time each day in which to eat your meals. In the 30 Day Challenge chapter, you will actually get to sample multiple types of Intermittent Fasting schedules. It's more about when you eat, as long as what you eat is healthy.

At this juncture

I would like to check in with you on any 1 thing which you have learnt of value.

Please share it with us on a review on amazon.

Thank you so much!

Chapter 5:
Dos and Don'ts for Intermittent Fasting

How are you doing so far? Lots of nutrition information, meal planning information, eating window information, and calorie information! It's a lot to take in. But just like starting a new class in school, those are the basics to Intermittent Fasting. They are a solid foundation that will help support your entire weight loss and health journey!

But, as you spend each day alternating between your eating windows and your times for Intermittent Fasting, you will also run into some obstacles here and there. That's why I've set up an entire list of 'Dos' and 'Don'ts' to help guide you in this chapter.

These are just a bunch of really helpful tips, and they provide the true keys to success when you decide to embark on this Intermittent Fasting lifestyle. How do you know what will bring you the results you need? How do you know what pitfalls to avoid, including many mistakes that I made! Here's your first don't: don't skip this chapter! Learn from me and do it the right way.

DO: Ease Into Your Intermittent Fasting

Breathe with me. Just breathe. In ... and out. Good!

It's easy to get overwhelmed when you start a new dieting plan.

Intermittent Fasting is not a race! I know you want to lose the weight quickly and have that goal number on the scale.

But please don't let impatience or eagerness cause you to bite off more than you can chew. Intermittent Fasting is going to give you the maximum success if you not only ease into it, but take your time to plan everything out. It's not just a diet; it's an entire lifestyle change. And it's only a lifestyle change that will benefit you if it's not rushed, if it really works the best with your schedule, and if you decide to put in the committed effort to make it work for you.

Patience is not just a virtue – it's also the key to losing lots of weight with Intermittent Fasting! Plan for your eating windows, prepare yourself for the hours of fasting, and spend as much time as you need finding the perfect eating window of time and the perfect meal plan schedule for you. Only then will you see the weight drop off … and you'll be a happier woman on each step of the journey, too.

DO: Stay Hydrated While Fasting

While you are abstaining from all calorie consumption during fasting, you want to make sure you stay well hydrated. In one of the below tips, I mention to keep a food diary. As part of your food diary, track how much water you are drinking as well. It's good to get in your eight glasses per day. Many of us don't realize that we're not drinking as much water as we should!

Water has so many other benefits, too. Your body is mostly made up of water, so every single cell needs it for optimum functions. To flavor plain water while you're Intermittently fasting, try adding a squeeze of lemon or a few berries to infuse a fruity flavor.

DO: Rest As Much As You Can

When was the last time you woke up refreshed from an amazing night's rest? It is one of the best feelings to be well rested. While you're Intermittent Fasting, your body is working hard to repair cells, help you lose weight, digest the healthy foods you've been eating, and perform all of its different functions – and it's best when your body is able to do these at night, while you are asleep.

So, get as much rest as you can while on the Intermittent Fasting plan. Sometimes making sure to sleep enough is even harder than going to the gym! But your mental alertness levels, your mood, your overall health, and your best weight will all be improved by a proper night's rest. How much sleep you need is completely individual! I need at least eight hours, while my husband seems to function well on only six or seven. Every person is different. Just make sure you're getting the optimum amount of rest for you.

As a bonus, the more you sleep, the faster those hours of fasting go by!

DO: Listen to Your Hunger Signals

In the previous couple of chapters, I mentioned the ghrelin hunger hormone a few times. Some women have a more difficult time fasting because this hormone has not adjusted to your fasting schedule yet. Give it time to ease into your shorter eating windows. If you have to start with a longer eating window, like ten hours, that is perfectly fine. Pay attention to your own ghrelin levels and when your hunger is the most ravenous.

It's a good idea to plan your eating windows around those peak hunger hormone times. This is all about working with your body's natural processes. Pay attention to your inner hunger signals. That is when you can eat your largest meal, with the highest calorie percentage. Then you can custom tailor your meal plan around that largest meal.

What about when you're hungry during times of fasting? You don't have to suffer through on sheer willpower. Within your first month or two of fasting, especially while you are in the 'testing the schedule' phase, you are allowed to have a very tiny amount of calories to see you through. This is especially helpful at night, if you're trying to fall asleep on an empty stomach. You can have a very small amount of nuts, one slice of cheese, half of a banana, half a glass of milk, or one other reduced serving of a food. This is not meant to satisfy your hunger, but to ease it. Only see these calories as a crutch.

As you spend more and more weeks Intermittent Fasting, the fasting will get easier. It also helps to eat plenty of protein, fiber-rich carbohydrates, and good, healthy fats to keep your tummy satiated between meals and eating windows.

DO: Meal Plan

Yes, yes, and more yes! You read about the sample meal plan templates in the previous chapter, so hopefully by now you're thinking about which one will fit best into your lifestyle.

Once you've decided on your first eating window meal plan template that works for your schedule, then start to calculate your individual calorie count requirements. From there, you can search online or in cookbooks for healthy recipes. Build healthy meals from the suggested ingredients list in Chapter 4. Then plan out your meals each week in your day planner or calendar.

Meal planning can be a pain. I mean, it's one more thing to do in my busy week! Meal planning takes a bit of time up front, but it saves you enormous amounts of time throughout the rest of your week. Since Intermittent Fasting is all about the clock, meal planning becomes that much more pertinent. It should be an essential part of your week. I'll talk more about Intermittent Fasting preparations in Chapter 7. It's so important!

DO: Keep a Food Diary

This is also really important. Every woman's eating and fasting journey is going to be unique, so there's no way you can compare mine to yours. I can give you plenty of tips, but I can't walk the road for you! A food diary not only keeps you accountable, but it also provides the most helpful and useful road map for the daily changes in your body.

Use a food diary to track:

- Your daily eating windows
- Your daily fasting times
- Your calorie percentages for each meal
- What you eat each day and the calorie counts
- How many glasses of water you drink each day
- How you feel each day
- What you weigh each week
- What ingredients to shop for
- And more!

While I am old school and like to keep my food diary in a paper planner, you can certainly find an app for your smartphone that works just as well. Make it personalized to your lifestyle, and you'll not only use it more, but it will be that much more helpful to you in the long run.

I've kept food diaries for years. It's amazing to look back and see not just how many pounds I've lost, but the daily steps it took to lose those pounds. Every weight loss journey takes weeks and months of time. A food diary helps you see all that time at a glance.

DON'T: Force Yourself to Fast

Fasting is not the same as starving or food deprivation. Far from it! Fasting is more similar to a resting period between meals. You are helping your body's digestive processes work better by fasting. You are not starving your body of nutrients or kicking your cells into more harmful things, like diabetic ketoacidosis, muscle deprivation, organ failure, bone weakening, or anything else. Those are serious conditions.

But have no fear. So, don't force yourself to fast, either. You don't have to fast to be healthy and lose weight. It's just one of the most natural ways to do so! If you are having difficulty with a particular fasting schedule or eating window, you can either cut back and only fast a few days a week instead of each day, or change your eating windows. To force your body to fast would only add more problems in the long run, so it's definitely not worth it!

On the other hand, if you enjoy fasting and you love both your eating window and your schedule, then by all means keep on doing what you're doing! If it isn't broke, don't fix it. Continue on the same path, use your food diary to monitor how you feel, and enjoy watching those pounds gradually and pretty effortlessly drop away. You'll also look and feel a whole lot better, too.

DON'T: Wing It

Yes, it's true. This is not an eating plan where you just wing it and hope for the best! It requires a lot of planning, consistency, and the ability to stick to the confines of the Intermittent Fasting schedule. That is why above I made the strong suggestion of meal planning. This is a diet where you are also watching the clock, so it's that important to make sure you're following a consistent routine. You need to be accountable to yourself.

So, once you have nailed down your ideal eating window / fasting schedule ratio, then please stick with it. Watch the clock, eat your meals on time, finish eating before the end of your eating window, plan for your one, two, or three meals per day, and just wash, rinse, repeat until you reach your weight loss goals.

This is definitely the kind of eating plan that works best with a consistent weekly schedule, but you can definitely do it if your life is crazy, too! That type of lifestyle just takes more planning.

If you are also following the Ketogenic Diet, which I'll chat about in Chapter 10, you shouldn't wing it with your Macros, either! Also, that is not a cheat day diet, where you can just jump off the wagon. It could knock you out of ketosis. So, when you're combining both the Keto Diet and Intermittent Fasting, you want to put in your due diligence to stick with it.

DON'T: Go This Alone

Even if you're doing Intermittent Fasting with a male partner or friend, his experience might not give you an accurate picture of this type of eating plan. So, find other women who are doing Intermittent Fasting! There are thousands of helpful gals out there who've had success, who've also gone through what you're going through, and they want to help you! Your feelings about how you live in your body each day are important. No one will understand that better than a fellow woman going through the same thing. She can also help hold you accountable to sticking to this!

So, in that light, don't try to go it alone with this Intermittent Fasting. Join an online forum or a dieting group in the real world. Talk about what you're going through. You might want to share your food diary, share your thoughts, and share your journey every step of the way. A blog could be a helpful place to just air your thoughts and experience with this. Any kind of outlet that helps you sort through your relationships between eating, fasting, and feelings is going to be so incredibly beneficial. You'll not just feel better when you finally achieve your weight loss goals. You will also have a better day to day experience!

DON'T: Be Afraid to Tweak Your Fasting Schedule

Life happens! It's okay to tweak and change your Intermittent Fasting schedule. If you become pregnant, are planning a huge life event like a wedding, have to take care of elderly parents, change jobs, move locations, suffer an emergency situation, or other big circumstances, that can certainly throw a wrench into your fasting schedule. There are just some times when being on an eating plan is too much work and one more thing to throw into an already overloaded schedule.

That's perfectly fine. Just give yourself the space and time to tweak your fasting schedule. You can move your eating window up by a few hours, go back to three meals instead of two (or drop down to two meals instead of three), or other changes. Just keep listening to your body, paying attention to your hunger hormones, and you'll still gain the benefits of fasting.

This has happened to me. I was on a two meal a day 6 hour fasting schedule, when I had an emergency situation happen in my husband's family. Our whole life seemed to stop and was put on hold for a month. My fasting schedule suddenly didn't work anymore, since our lives were so topsy turvy. I went down to OMAD and ate it in the morning, so I could attend and help out for the rest of the day without worrying about getting myself lunch or dinner. I could just be there in the hospital. After everything had smoothed over and I'd gone back to normal, I spent a few days tweaking my fasting schedule and increasing back to the 6 hour eating window.

So, if something happens to you, just know that your fasting schedule is not set in stone. It's there for you to customize depending on how your life is going.

Do the Intermittent Fasting Your Way

Every woman's life is different. We all have our own lives with our families, friends, work, home, hobbies, and other things that fill up our time. Intermittent Fasting is the most flexible eating plan you'll ever be on, so take advantage of it and make it work for you. These tips in this chapter prevent most of the issues with Intermittent Fasting for women and are helpful signposts along the way as you navigate through your own dieting journey.

Oh, and one last do for you: show off your progress! Take those awesome 'before' and 'after' pictures that are so fun to see and share on social media. Take a picture of yourself each month and watch those pounds come off.

You'll have so much success just by using Intermittent Fasting!

Chapter 6:
Being a Mom on Intermittent Fasting

Hi there fellow moms!

Now, this is a chapter you won't see in a lot of Intermittent Fasting books, especially those written by men.

But for me to not include my husband and children on my Intermittent Fasting journey would be so incredibly difficult, that I wouldn't be able to do it! I'd be doomed from the start. In fact, a huge part of my own personal success has happened because I took my family into account, too.

So, this is a book that is for the mothers who want to lose weight. If you don't have children, you can certainly get a lot of great tips from this chapter, too. I'm a mom who has committed to this lifestyle and not only changed my body for myself, but changed it in a better way that benefits my entire family. I feel better, and a happy mom equals a happier home life. That's for sure!

The moms who commit to this and make a change for both yourselves and your children are super happy. You can read many success stories online.

You want to be happier for your sons and daughters, too. They mean the absolute world to you, and it's the easiest thing in the world to put them first. First, meaning above yourself.

But what about your own health? You want to live for your kids. You want to change the future of what you see for yourself. You've probably already tried different things to lose the weight, but the failures have piled up.

How about doing something different this time? You will feel better trying Intermittent Fasting than any other kind of dieting or eating or fitness plan. Let's pick a diet you can sustain for the rest of your life. That also means starting slow with workouts, too.

So, whether you're trying to lose weight after giving birth, want to get back to your former size before children, or just want to have more energy, vitality, and a better overall outlook with your husband and kids, I'm here to help you succeed on Intermittent Fasting!

Balance vs. Busy Life

If every woman who's heard the term "work-life balance" was paid a dollar, we'd all be millionaires! It seems that no matter how hard we try, we can't be super moms and have it all for longer than a few months before becoming exhausted and burning out. You have to look out for your kids, help out around the house, feed those hungry mouths, have your own full-time job (or multiple jobs), and somehow have enough time to follow an eating plan, let alone have success on it?

No wonder so many of us have been stuck in 'yo-yo' dieting purgatory for years.

Intermittent Fasting has so many extraordinary benefits for even the busiest lifestyle. In fact, the busier my life gets, the easier it becomes for me to fast and lose weight. Yep, you read that right:

The busier your life gets, the easier Intermittent Fasting becomes.

What kind of magical statement is that? I'm not surprised you're skeptical.

The reason Intermittent Fasting is the ultimate eating plan for your busy lifestyle is because you customize it to work around all that hectic craziness.

As you read in Chapter 4, there are a bunch of sample meal plan templates for you to choose from. Each of them will work beautifully if you just follow them every day. Each of them is a path towards losing weight.

The only thing you have to do is pick one of those templates and stick to it. You can also definitely tweak and customize your schedule if life throws you a curveball. I talked more about that in the last chapter.

Doing Intermittent Fasting is actually easier than if you weren't fasting! Do you have a certain busy time of day where it's just impossible to prep and cook a meal? Then add that time of day to your fasting period, and set up your eating windows around it.

For me, this is the morning. I need to wake my kids up, get them ready for school, and make sure they have a packed lunch. I already meal planned to make sure that their breakfasts are ready to go, but it's just too much to also try and eat something for myself at the same time. They finish breakfast quickly and get out the door. I break my fast with my first meal of the day two hours after they leave, which is plenty of time to prep and cook that meal. I've grown used to this schedule, so I'm not even hungry in the morning until that meal time comes around.

Pretty simple. It also takes all the guesswork out of trying to balance your life.

Life is full of ups and downs, but even more so when you have kids. Embrace the ups and downs. Add Intermittent Fasting and your eating windows to your life. They will help you work with your crazy schedule – and before you know it, the weight will start to drop off.

Planning Mom Equals Happy Mom

As a mom, do you know what really helps both my sanity and my weight loss?

Having a plan. Specifically, my meal plan each week. I actually plan out two meal plans into one large meal plan: my own Intermittent Fasting meal plan, and my kids' meals. I don't cook entirely separate meals from my kids, but I make sure that they have their own healthy things that they're eating. I include what they want each week as part of their meal plan, too.

When I'm done meal planning for my kids, I post their meals on the fridge each week, so that they can see it. Do I still get asked what's for dinner? Yep, sometimes! My kids can forget. But I pretty much always have the answer right there on my fridge.

In addition to just writing down what we're having for meals in my family, I also include grocery shopping lists. That makes it super easy to shop for exactly what I need for those meals!

I'm a mom who plans, and boy, am I a happy mom because of it!

So, for my fellow moms out there, I urge you to plan out not just your own Intermittent Fasting meals, but those for your children as well.

Meal planning is definitely one weekly task of mine that I actually look forward to! That is because it saves so much time in the long run. I know that the hour or two that it takes to sit down with your kids on a weekend afternoon to plan out the meals and shopping lists for ingredients is time that will not just be saved, but will also pay me back in pounds of weight loss.

Remember that:

A Meal Plan Saves Time and Pays You Back in Weight Loss!

The same goes for you, too!

Eating for You, Eating for Kids!

What kinds of recipes are going to go on your meal plans for the adults and the kids in the house?

Children like to eat simpler, blander meals than adults do. Their taste buds are more sensitive, and they like to eat things that have lots of sugars, salts, and creamy or crunchy textures. They will gladly reach for the junk food! Kid fave food choices include ice cream, pizza, burgers and fries, hot dogs, popcorn, potato chips, chicken tenders with dipping sauce, macaroni and cheese, spaghetti with meatballs, and candy. While you can find some healthy versions of these foods, they are definitely not going to help you with your weight loss goals. It's time for more greens and more proteins!

When you're putting together your meal plan, don't forget to slowly but steadily shift away from unhealthy recipes and choose healthier ones instead. Also, try to include common ingredients in both meal plans that will appeal to both kid and adult palates.

What kinds of foods are great for both kids and you?

- All those wonderful healthy vegetables listed back in Chapter 4. You can roast vegetables, put them into soups, add them to a wrap, stir-fry them, make salads, or puree them to serve with a main entrée course of meat or fish.
- Fruits are also delicious for both kids and adults. Apples, bananas, oranges, berries, and sliced melon are usual favorites.
- Fill your kids' bellies with a good amount of proteins for growing muscles, healthy brain function, and energy. You'll both enjoy chicken, turkey, ham, pork, beef, fish, and different kinds of seafood.
- Kids love cheese, and moms do, too! Look for yummy full fat cheeses and other healthy dairy products.

- Kids can really enjoy fiber rich carbohydrates, like whole grain bread, oatmeal, canned beans, barley, and other options.
- Both you and your kids can include nuts and seeds in your diets.

Search online for more kid friendly and all natural breakfast, lunch, and dinner options. As with the adult options, stay away from packaged foods and anything stuffed with chemicals, artificial flavors, colors, and especially sweeteners. Kids' smaller bodies are especially susceptible to spikes in blood sugar, which you will definitely see as they go crazy from a sugar rush!

I don't know about your kids, but mine love eating the same ten or fifteen meal choices over and over. They don't seem to get bored! I introduce new foods to them every couple of weeks, just for a bit of variety. It also seems like, since they have a lot of input into their own meal plans, that they understand the whole process of grocery shopping, cooking, and eating a lot more. They are interested in it, and they actually help me out quite a bit.

These are wonderful life lessons to help teach your kids. Your weight loss and health journey is a part of their lives, too. Maybe they will grow up understanding the essential links between diets, fitness, health, and weight loss. That is a valuable thing to learn!

Exercising and Intermittent Fasting as a Mom

When you're a busy mom with a packed schedule, exercising seems a like a whole lot of extra work that you just wouldn't be able to fit in. Unless you involve your kids with you, it takes time away from them, too. Who is going to watch them while you work out at the gym?

It is also both natural and normal to be intimidated, scared, or otherwise averse to going to the gym.

I know I was.

I had plenty of really good reasons why I wasn't getting any exercise, but most of them had to do with fear. I was afraid of going to the gym and looking like an idiot, sweating profusely in front of others. Maybe that is a silly fear, but it kept me from exercising – and it kept me from losing the weight I wanted to.

So, I just started out with Intermittent Fasting, eating windows, and choosing healthier ingredients. I put exercising on the back burner. After a month, I'd gotten used to fasting, I was much more comfortable with my eating windows, I'd already lost ten pounds, and I finally felt like it was time to add exercise to the mix. I wanted to up my weight loss, too!

But I really had no idea where or how to start. My favorite exercise has always been walking. I love to walk everywhere. Would walking be exercise enough to shed pounds while fasting? I had no idea, but it was a question I wanted to answer with a yes!

I began a daily walking routine of just fifteen minutes. That is once around the block of my neighborhood. After a few days, I increased it to thirty minutes by walking twice around the block. I kept up that routine for several weeks, and I was shocked at my results. I mean, all I was doing was walking twice around the block! But that was when the weight really started to drop off. My body also felt better, I felt lighter inside, and my legs felt better, too.

That's when I finally bit the bullet and bought a gym membership. I was very scared the first few times! I just tentatively started on the treadmill and walked for thirty minutes, increasing my incline. But you know what? After that first week, it definitely got easier. The days passed, and I enjoyed the treadmill. It took me about a month to get used to just going to the gym as part of my daily routine. My kids sometimes joined me, too! They loved using the equipment.

Gradually, I went from the treadmill to using other machines at the gym, like the stationary bikes and rowing machines. Then, I started using kettlebells as part of weight training.

Nowadays, I'm a much more confident gym goer! I work out for thirty minutes each day, using a combination of different machines and the kettlebells. I still get a bit trepidatious, but then I remind myself of all the pounds of weight I've lost because I added exercise to my Intermittent Fasting. I also look better than I have in years. I feel stronger, leaner, and fitter.

I hope my story can give you some idea of how you can add exercise to your eating plan, too!

Just start with a simple walking routine. If you can't get to the gym, then you can buy a treadmill. Just fifteen minutes of walking today, to start. Even with kids, you can do this!

Build a Support System

Any kind of diet plan while you're a mom can feel like its own upward hill climb when you're living in a house full of people who aren't doing what you're doing.

So, it's absolutely essential that you have a support system. You need girlfriends and relatives and other Intermittent Fasting women to talk to! You need to be able to rant about a difficult day, vent about the rocky patches, and just share what you're feeling and what you're thinking with like-minded, compassionate souls.

The women who have experienced the most successful weight loss journeys have had support to do it. You can find this support system online or through reaching out to other women in your community. These women will help cheer you on, hold you accountable, and you can support their goals, too.

Don't forget to include yourself in your support system, too. Support your own weight loss goals and fitness goals. Ask for help around the house when you need it. Teach your kids how to be there with you along the way as you get healthier.

The more support you have, the more successful you will be!

Your Body is For You

What's great about Intermittent Fasting, is that I have done so much of the nutrition research for you! If you'd like, you can go back to Chapter 3 and read all about the actual science behind what is going on in your body. And yes, all of that stuff is true even after you have had children! Your body doesn't magically stop processing nutrients the way it did before you got pregnant. So, that's good news! That means this will work.

While you may be inspired to get healthy for your husband or your children, ultimately, they don't live inside your body. They don't know how you feel each day, they are different people with their own trials and tribulations, and they aren't going to take the same journey as you.

Just like any journey, this Intermittent Fasting one begins with the proper preparations. That is what you will read about in the next chapter!

Chapter 7:
Easy Guide to Starting
Intermittent Fasting

Let's say you want to go on a two tropical vacation to the Caribbean. You can't wait to have fun in the sun. Would you leave the house without packing for your trip? Of course not! You need your bathing suit, sunscreen, beach towels, clothes, makeup, and other stuff to take with you. I also never go on vacation without at least having a packing list!

Think of this chapter as similar to a travel packing list. We are going to go over absolutely everything you need to know to prepare yourself for Intermittent Fasting. The next chapter is my favorite in the book and has your 30 Day Challenge. But before we get started, it's time to get ready!

Prepping for the Journey

I want you to go through each step of preparing for your Intermittent Fasting 30 Day Challenge. Take as much time as you need, but the whole process shouldn't take longer than a week or so. It's okay to fit this into your busy schedule!

By now, you have read through many aspects of Intermittent Fasting, and you are probably starting to realize this is definitely an eating plan and fasting plan that has as much to do with mental preparations as any other endeavor. You are going to get your mind ready to go as much as anything physical that you'll do. Your mindset should be one of openness, curiosity, excitement, and be flexible enough to handle any and all challenges that come your way.

Got it?

Okay, good. Now, we will move on to a few of your personal numbers that I want you to calculate before we go about finding recipes and meals.

Setting an Eating Window:

If you have not done so already, go back to Chapter 4 and read over the sample meal plan and fasting plan templates. Choose the amount of time that you'd like for your eating window. You will also pick whether you'd like to eat one, two, or three meals per day. Meals usually last about one to two hours. Then calculate when your eating window will begin and when it will end.

Write all of this information below:

My Eating Window Lasts _____ Hours

Eating Window Start Time: _____ am / pm

Eating Window End Time: _____ am / pm

Number of Meals Per Day: _____ meals

Meal #1 Time: _____ am / pm to _____ am / pm

Meal #2 Time: _____ am / pm to _____ am / pm

Meal #3 Time: _____ am / pm to _____ am / pm

Okay, great! Remember that this information is flexible, and you can change it at any point. This will be personalized to you. I like to write my eating window information on the first page of my food diary. That helps me remember it while I am going about my day.

Setting Your Calorie Requirements:

Next, is to figure out your calorie requirements. You can find that in an online calorie calculator. Then, we will divvy up those calories amongst your meals. Refer back to the sample meal plan templates in Chapter 4 to get a better idea of what percentages work best with either one meal, two meals, or three meals. Those percentages should all add up to 100%.

Write all of this information below:

Calories Per Day: _____

Meal #1 is _____ % of my daily calories = _____ calories

Meal #2 is _____ % of my daily calories = _____ calories

Meal #3 is _____ % of my daily calories = _____ calories

Great! Now you know exactly how many calories to consume in each meal. Those calories are going to be a mixture of the healthy food ingredients you read about in Chapter 4 as well.

Setting Goals:

You have your baseline eating window times, your meal plan times, and your calorie counts. Now it's time to set your goals. You get thirty days' worth of Intermittent Fasting days in the next chapter to get through. So, what are your weight loss goals for the next four weeks? I break my weight loss goals down into smaller five pound or ten pound milestones. That way, I don't get overwhelmed by lots of weight to lose. I just focus on losing the next five pounds.

I also want you to think about your exercise goals, too. That is largely about setting up a gym going or home exercise routine of various activities that will help shed the pounds and strengthen your body at the same time.

Fill in your goals in the spaces below:

Overall Weight Loss Goal: _____ pounds

Current Weight: _____ pounds

Goal Weight: _____ pounds

First Weight Loss Milestone: _____ pounds lost in _____ weeks

Second Weight Loss Milestone: _____ pounds lost in _____ weeks

Third Weight Loss Milestone: _____ pounds lost in _____ weeks

Exercise Goal: _____ minutes per day and _____ days per week

Exercise Start Time: _____ am / pm

Exercise End Time: _____ am / pm

Exercise Routine: _____

I include my goals right on the front page of my food diary. They help keep me motivated, and it's amazing to see how far I've come just by using Intermittent Fasting on a regular basis.

With your numbers prepped, ready to go, and written down in an app or food diary or place where you can see them pretty much each day, you know where you start. The journey begins with finding out where you are today – and these numbers tell you that in great detail.

Finding Recipes and Meals

Here is the fun part of any eating plan – finding recipes and meal ideas to go into your meal plan! Whether you are eating one, two, or three meals a day, you have your calorie counts for each of those meals. Now, it's just a matter of finding delicious foods and flavors that will satisfy your nutritional requirements.

There are just certain types of foods that we love to have with our meals each day. If you think of your meals in terms of categories, that makes it easier. Check out my ideas below:

Meal 1: Breakfast

Whether you're eating two or three meals per day, typical breakfast food options are really popular. These are actually my absolute favorite foods. I could eat breakfast for dinner, too! Breakfast foods are also popular with kids, if you're a mom. Here are some breakfast food options you will love to have to help you when you literally break your fast.

- Smoothies, especially ones with an avocado or coconut milk base to give you plenty of good fats to start your day. Stick in a handful of fresh baby spinach or kale to sneak veggies into your diet.
- Egg dishes, like baked eggs, scrambled eggs, frittatas, quiche, and omelets stuffed with veggies and cheeses.
- Meat options include bacon, sausage, or even steak.
- Breakfast bowls are popular, so have fun searching for ones that contain healthy ingredients like vegetables and different herbs or spices.
- For breakfast beverages, you can have milk, low sugar orange juice, low sugar fruit juice like strawberry banana, coffee, or tea. Bulletproof coffee, which has been enhanced with good fats like butter, is a popular and tasty option, too.

Meal 2: Lunch

Most of us eat lunch at work, and you only get an hour at the most. So, I often take last night's dinner as leftovers for lunch! My favorite lunch options are either hearty and filling soups or salads with plenty of toppings. If you are eating just two meals a day and lunch is your biggest meal, you might want to check out the dinner ideas and have supper for lunch instead. Here are other lunch options:

- Home made soups, usually made in the crockpot to make them easier. Popular ones include chicken noodle, beef stew, chunky minestrone, and hearty vegetable. Kids really love soup, too.
- A hearty salad that starts with a base of greens like Romaine lettuce, baby spinach, and chopped kale. Top with more sliced fresh veggies like mushrooms, bell pepper, tomato, red onion, carrots, cucumbers, or celery. Then add pre-cooked chicken, beef, turkey, or ham. I also add a handful of cheese like Feta or shredded cheddar, and a sprinkling of crunchy extras

like seeds and nuts. For dressing, I like many different flavors to add variety. Buy all natural salad dressings that have an olive oil or dairy base, limited chemicals, and no added sugars.

- Healthy sandwiches with whole grain bread, mayo or mustard or pesto, and then plenty of cheese, proteins like chicken or ham or bacon, and lots of veggies. Serve alongside pickles or fresh vegetables with hummus to dip.
- Lunch beverages include milk, green or fruit or herbal teas, low sugar fruit juice, or ice water with lemon.

Meal 3: Dinner

Dinners, also known as your last meal or third meal, usually feature the majority of your daily calories. They are built around one major hearty protein choice like chicken, beef, pork, ham, fish, or seafood. This protein is usually served alongside a cooked or roasted vegetable like carrots, onions, potatoes, broccoli, cauliflower, or mushrooms. You can also expand your palate by choosing foods from around the world for dinner. What else could be for dinner?

- Find healthy recipes for your family's favorite ten dinner options.
- Try a new dinner option every two weeks. Pick a country with different flavors and try to incorporate that dish into the menu. Popular options include French food, Thai food, Indian food, Greek food, Spanish food, and Japanese food.
- Substitute brown rice, wild rice, barley, quinoa, or whole wheat for rice, corn, and white flour carbohydrates.
- Dinner beverage options are ice water with lemon, milk, or the occasional glass of wine.

These meal options are just here to give you an idea of the different things you could eat for your one, two, or three meals each day. On a two meal a day plan, you could have breakfast and dinner, with no lunch foods, lunch and dinner with no breakfast foods, or breakfast and lunch with no dinner foods. This eating plan really is customizable to your life!

It's more about when you eat. As long as you choose healthy, natural ingredients like those above, you will do just fine!

Creating Your Weekly Meal Plan

Meal planning is made a lot easier when you have all the meal ideas and recipes from the last step ready to go. I have a folder on my computer that contains all of my recipes for each meal. That makes it a lot easier to just add those to my weekly meal plan and much easier to create grocery lists, too.

I thought I'd share my weekly meal plan template with you. I eat two meals a day. I type this up on the computer, then print it out and put it on the fridge each week for my kids to see it, too. That way, everyone knows what we're eating when!

Date: _____

Meal 1 at 12:00 pm.

      Recipe: _____

      Calories: _____

Meal 2 at 4:00 pm.

      Recipe: _____

      Calories: _____

Kids' Dinner: _____

Feel free to customize this sample daily meal plan template! I have a 6 hour eating window and eat just two meals a day. Are you eating three meals a day instead? Then add the extra lines for the third meal. Are you eating just one meal a day? Then include all the recipes and calories for the foods in that one meal. You can play around with this basic idea to really make your meal plan your own.

I also have kids, so they get their own dinner option. That way, I know what to make for them, if I have to make something separately. Usually, though, I eat what they're eating! I do make healthy versions of foods, so both Mom and the kids are happy and healthy.

The Kitchen Equipment You'll Need

Do you need to purchase anything fancy and special to make delicious Intermittent Fasting meals?

Not unless you really want to! I am able to make all kinds of delicious items using basic kitchen equipment like my 12" cast iron skillet, several saucepans in different sizes, three large cookie sheets with a cooling rack, a high-speed blender for making smoothies, a large crock pot or slow cooker, and a food processor. Instant Pots have recently become popular, so you could get one in a larger family size to cut down the amount of time to make many crock pot dishes.

Whichever recipes you've decided to make that go with your calorie counts and your personal tastes, they can usually be made using the above equipment. It helps to have everything washed, cleaned, and ready to go as part of your overall Intermittent Fasting preparations!

Creating a Grocery List

Meal planning makes creating grocery lists so easy! With your seven days' worth of meals in front of you, you can quickly rifle through the fridge, cupboards, and freezer to see what you need to stock up on.

I created a grocery list template on my computer that has all the food categories of items to restock. I tend to buy a lot of pantry and cupboard items in bulk that have a long shelf life.

Then, I spend about an hour each week purchasing the fresher ingredients for that week's meals. After doing this for several weeks, you'll find that grocery shopping is a breeze. You will also discover that you keep purchasing the same items over and over. That is a good thing! It means you're committed to only buying healthier ingredients, and that you're not tempted to put something in your cart that could slow down your weight loss.

Remember Gin's Golden Rule of Grocery Shopping for Weight Loss:

If It Doesn't Go in the Cart, it Can't Go in Your House and it Won't Get Eaten!

Weight loss begins at the grocery store, lovely ladies. Stick to your healthy shopping list, and you will stick to your weight loss goals.

Here are the grocery store categories that correspond to most grocery stores:

Produce & Fresh Herbs:

- In the produce section is where you'll get your fresh vegetables and fruits for the week.
- You can buy fresh garlic and fresh herbs in this section as well.

Meat & Seafood:

- Buy the best quality proteins, fish, and seafoods that you can afford, since they won't have as many harmful ingredients.
- You can purchase meats in bulk, portion it out into plastic bags, and store them in the freezer.

Eggs & Dairy:

- In the cheese section at your store, you can find all the cheeses to add to your grocery cart.
- The milk, eggs, butter, yogurt, and other dairy items are often kept in a different part of the store. I replenish my dairy items all the time, since we eat them so much in my house!

Nuts, Seeds, and Baking:

- I buy nuts and seeds in bulk and store them in airtight containers in my pantry cupboards.
- Shop in the baking aisle for your baking ingredients. I like to bake some home made healthy treats like crackers, granola bars, and healthy cookies.

Herbs, Spices, and Condiments:

- Dried herbs (fresh herbs go in the produce category) and dried spices. I keep a fully stocked herb and spice cabinet. I sometimes visit different ethnic markets to find herbs and spices that are inexpensive, unusual, or distinctive.
- Condiments include oils, vinegars, barbecue sauce, soy sauce, mayo, ketchup, and similar. Check labels, since these are packaged goods and frequently have too many harmful chemicals.

Frozen Section:

- The frozen section has a lot of packaged foods, so read your labels carefully here.
- I buy frozen vegetables, some frozen meats, and occasionally a small tub of healthy frozen yogurt.

Other:

- Coffee, wine, tea, and other items that don't fit into any other categories go in this part of my grocery list.

You can customize this list to fit your own stores. I sometimes create separate grocery lists for buying items online, at different markets, and at different stores.

Cooking Your Meals

Fasting for at least fourteen hours per day gives you some extra time to prep and cook the recipes for the meals on your meal plan. It's sometimes the prep work that takes the most time, so I cut down on that and save time by slicing vegetables and storing them in sealed plastic bags in the fridge. I also like to pre cook favorite foods like chicken breasts, bacon, and beef ahead of time. That way, it's easy to combine those ingredients with others and make dishes.

While you are planning out your meals for your eating windows, you might want to include the cooking times. It's all about preparing yourself for the 30 Day Intermittent Fasting Challenge to come!

Preparing for Fasting

What about your actual fasting times in between meals? What kind of preparations should you put in place for those?

Water and Hydration

Prepare for your fast by drinking plenty of water! You are also allowed to have water, perhaps with some fresh lemon slices, to sip on throughout the fast, too. It might help to stock up on plastic water bottles, a plastic water jug for the fridge, and any other items you will need to remind yourself to keep drinking water.

Having Tiny Snacks

Throughout your first few weeks trying Intermittent Fasting, it helps to have a few small snacks available during those fasting periods. It helps to get your body over the 'hump' of changing your metabolism, adjusting to fasting, and encouraging your cells to seek fat from your adipose cells instead of relying on incoming glucose. These tiny snacks should be no more than 80 calories at the absolute most. By the third week, your body will have grown used to Intermittent Fasting, and you will no longer need to have any calories for those periods of time between your eating windows.

Longer Fasting

What about preparing for longer fasting periods? In the 30 Day Challenge, I include a 24 hour fasting day. For those longer fasts, you would want to eat all of your calories like normal the day before the fast, but abstain from exercising that day, the day of the fast, and the day after as well. You would also want to break your fast with a well balanced and good protein rich meal that has plenty of essential vitamins and nutrients. I'll talk more about that with the longer fasting in the next chapter.

Support System

If you read the chapter about being a mom on Intermittent Fasting, you read about putting a support system in place. This is another preparation to do before you start fasting. If you haven't already, find an Intermittent Fasting community online and reach out to other women who are doing this along with you! They can give you real life examples of what they're going through and answer more specific questions about their journeys. It's very helpful!

Fasting Activities

Before you begin Intermittent Fasting, you might want to think about what kinds of activities you would do during your fasting periods. I was surprised to discover that, since I had cut out a meal, I now had that free time. If you already have a busy lifestyle, this is definitely one of the perks! You would simply be able to fill the new time with more things in your schedule. But it does help to add more activities into your life during your fasting times.

Tracking Your Progress

As part of preparing for Intermittent Fasting, you want to find the ideal tracking method for you that will be a helpful resource for collecting and writing down your own 'data' about this weight loss plan. You want to treat yourself to a nice paper food diary or find a great app for your smartphone that can be a resource to help you.

There are so many parts of Intermittent Fasting to track! Here are just a few ideas you could put into the diary:

- Track your weight loss goals
- Track how you feel and what you're experiencing each day of Intermittent Fasting
- Track what you eat and the calorie counts
- Track the water that you're drinking each day
- Track the exercise routine that you have chosen
- Track any new recipes you find
- Track how a new healthy recipe tasted
- Track grocery shopping

I am in love with tracking! I do like data and numbers. They give me a much clearer picture of what is really going on in my weight loss journey than just my own memories and experiences of it.

Tracking is also a way of honoring your commitment to changing your body for the better. You are putting how you feel in your body first! Your record of this experience is just confirmation of how much strength and courage it takes to not just try something new, but to believe that it will work. That is inspirational!

Tomorrow is When We Begin

Okay, you are now completely prepped and ready to begin the 30 Day Challenge of Intermittent Fasting! You have accomplished a lot, and you haven't even begun your first day of fasting yet!

Let's see what you did:

- You have found your first eating window in which to begin
- You've decided how many meals you'll eat
- You looked up your daily calorie requirements
- You divvied up those calories amongst your meals
- You set your weight loss and exercise goals
- You found recipes and ideas for eating
- You made an amazing meal plan based on those recipes
- You also created grocery lists that have healthy ingredients
- You stocked your kitchen with equipment to make your meals
- You have what you need to see you through your fasts – water bottle, snacks, etc.
- You have a tracking method, either a food diary or an app

That is a lot, but you will need it all throughout the next thirty days.

The final thing to do to before starting tomorrow? Take a selfie! Make sure that you take a picture of yourself as you are now. Are you ready to work towards changing your body and having a whole new you after fasting?

Then let's get started.

Chapter 8:
Intermittent Fasting 30 Day Challenge

Last chapter gave you so many tools to prepare you for this challenge! I hope you have all of them in place, because today is the day to get started.

We have laid the groundwork for a successful first month spent Intermittent Fasting.

This is the nuts and bolts chapter, that shows you exactly what a life of steady Intermittent Fasting looks like. This is a 30 Day Challenge that you can begin at any time, when it is most convenient for you. I encourage you to just read this entire chapter from start to finish before you begin. That will give you an overall view of the whole thing.

Then, you just start on Day One!

Fasting Foundation for Success

I personally designed this 30 Day Challenge for a complete beginning to start on Day One. We're going to split this into three different sections of 10 days each:

- Beginner – 10 days of skipped meals, getting used to Intermittent Fasting, and finding the perfect eating window that works for you.
- Intermediate – 10 days of locking in your eating window, then getting your recommended calories in that eating window.
- Advanced – 10 days of more advanced Intermittent Fasting, including your first 24-hour fast, as well as a 48-hour fast.

What's awesome about these three levels is that after you've completed the 30 Day Challenge, you can certainly go back to the Beginner or Intermediate section – and stay there for months at a time. Intermittent Fasting is meant to be a lifelong eating and fasting plan, so it's safe for you to do that.

As a quick note, just keep in mind that this guide is just one way to incorporate Intermittent Fasting into your life. As always with this way of eating, you are more than welcome to change it and customize it to suit your needs. If you're confident in your ability to start with small eating windows and you'll be fine with that, you're more than welcome to skip ahead to the Intermediate section.

It's not so much where you start – it's the fact that you will start! I also want you to enjoy yourself throughout your time spent Intermittent Fasting. This is an eating plan you can stick with for your whole life! So, it's worth it to take that extra step to enjoy each day of it.

Ready to get started? Let's go to the Beginner section.

Beginner Intermittent Fasting

Day 1

Day 1 of our 30 Day Intermittent Fasting Challenge has begun. Today is when you are going to ease slowly into this and try to eat your first day within a large eating window. If your ultimate goal is to eat within six hours, that is too much change too fast. It could possibly derail your plans and goals in the long run. You are advised to start out with an eating window of ten hours, which would give you a fasting time of fourteen hours. The ratio is 10:14. I also suggest you start out with a three meal a day schedule, instead of two meals. There will be plenty of time to drop back to eating fewer meals. But the slower you begin this, the more time your body will have to adjust.

You can start your 10 hour eating window at any time you like and whichever time works best in your schedule. Let's say you start it at 8:00 in the morning. Counting forward ten hours, that would give you until 6:00 pm at the latest to eat all of your calories for the day. When 6:00 pm rolls around, cease all food until tomorrow except for water.

If you have not already done so, today would also be the ideal time to plan out your meals for the rest of the week, find recipes using healthy ingredients, and go for a grocery shop to stock up your kitchen. For those who already have an exercise routine, it's perfectly fine to continue that today. But if you don't, that's okay, too! We'll include exercise after you've gotten used to the fasting schedule.

At the end of the day, take out your food diary. Track and record your eating window, what you ate today, and your overall experience. You will do this each day, and it's an excellent habit that will help you lose more weight than you've dreamed of!

Day 2

Great, you got through Day 1! How did that go? Hopefully you had a good experience with it. Today is when you are going to repeat your 10 hour eating window / 14 hour fasting routine. Do it at the same time you did the 10 hours yesterday. Then gently break your fast by eating a healthy meal. Continue on your meal plan until the end of your 10 hour eating window, then stop and begin the fasting part of the cycle.

Did you have any difficulty sustaining a 14 hour fast between yesterday and today? Since we're starting with a larger eating window, fourteen hours is a much shorter time to fast. Track and record in your food diary what you ate today and how your first official Intermittent Fasting period went.

Day 3

If Day 2 was fine and you enjoyed it, then repeat your 10 hour eating window / 14 hour fasting time today. As the days go by, it becomes easier and easier to get into the routine of eating and fasting. How are you doing with your calorie counting, cooking, and eating your meals? Eating all of your daily calorie requirements within a 10 hour window is pretty doable. Are you hungry at all during the fasting periods? Many of us are used to snacking or nibbling on something whenever we feel like it. So, to deliberately fast can seem a little odd at first. Keep pursuing it.

Track and record what you ate today and how your fasting is going for you.

Day 4

Another repeat day of the 10 hour eating window / 14 hour fasting period. Follow your meal plan, eat your meals at the correct times, and eat all of your calories within the 10 hour window.

As your body gets used to fasting, your hunger might start to drop off a bit. You'll also notice during the day when you're the hungriest. Remember that your ghrelin hunger hormones are at their highest around noon, and then taper off as you get closer to 8:00 pm at night. As long as you're eating healthy and following your recipes to cook good meals, you're on the right track.

Track and record what you ate today and how your fasting is going. Are you struggling with hunger or other minor health issues like headaches? Or, has your body adapted well to this so far? Write down your answer.

Day 5

Another repeat day of the 10 hour eating window / 14 hour fasting period. Keep following the meal plan, having your meals at appropriate times, eating all your calories before the end of the eating window, and ceasing all calorie consumption after the ten hour window ends.

Throughout the first five days of this challenge is when you have the most flexibility to tweak your eating window times. For example, you might have discovered that starting your eating window early in the day doesn't work, because you're ravenously hungry during your fasting times. So, you can move it to later in the day. You have options.

Track and record what you ate today and how the fasting is going.

Day 6

Now that you've been Intermittent Fasting for five days, you should have locked in a good eating window by this time. That's the time that works best for you, your family, and your schedule, too. You've also started to grow used to watching the clock, eating meals at certain times, and tracking your calories. I personally love the routine-ness of this diet, where I can just eat at the same times each day. You might like it, too!

As for today, we are going to do one final 10 hour eating window / 14 hour fasting time before we start shortening our eating window tomorrow. After today, you really shouldn't play around with moving your eating window earlier or later. Consistency and routine will be the best for weight loss! Track and record what you ate today.

Day 7

Congrats – you got to the end of your first week of 10 hour Intermittent Fasting! That wasn't so bad, was it? Once you get a hang of the routine, it becomes easier to incorporate it into your lifestyle. Are you doing well during the fasting times? Drinking plenty of water? If you needed to supplement one of the 14 hour periods with a tiny snack, that's perfectly fine.

Today is when you will drop your eating times back one hour. That means your eating window has shortened from 10 hours to 9 hours. Adjust your meal times accordingly. You are welcome to still eat the three meals, or to try just two larger meals per day if you're feeling like you've got the hang of this. You will also increase your fasting time from 14 hours to 15 hours. So, if your eating window for six days has ended at 6:00 pm at night, it now ends at 5:00 pm.

Track and record what you ate today and your new eating window of 9 hours.

Day 8

Day 8's meal times and 9-hour eating window is a repeat from yesterday. You fasted for 15 hours between yesterday and today, so you're starting to push your body a little bit more than just fasting for 14 hours. Drink water, get some rest, and just concentrate on eating all of your calories within the 9 hours. It seems like a lot of time, but it goes by quickly! Every woman I know, including myself, is a busy gal.

Day 8 is also an excellent time to readjust your meal plan, find new recipes for the next week, and go shopping for those ingredients to restock your kitchen.

Track and record what you ate today, your new eating window, and your calories.

Day 9

The 9 hour eating window repeats again today. Eat your meals at their adjusted times. You fasted 15 hours between yesterday and today. You have been Intermittent Fasting for over a week now. If you would like to begin an exercise routine while still in this first ten-day beginner part of the challenge, then today would be the perfect time to do it. Don't push yourself too much. Just increase your heart rate doing an exercise for about 15 to 20 minutes.

Track and record what you ate today, your fasting experience, and the exercise you've started doing.

Day 10

Today is the final day of the beginner section of this 30 Day Challenge. You started out with a 10 hour eating window, dropped back to 9 hours, increased your fasting, learned how to time meals and eat them within your windows, and perhaps also tried some exercising, too.

For today, you can continue on your 9 hour eating window / 15 hour fasting times. It's the final day of this schedule, since we're going to drop back one more hour tomorrow. Continue with your light exercise regimen, too.

Today would be a great time to weigh yourself. Have you lost any weight yet? A healthy weight loss schedule is up to two pounds per week. The combination of healthy eating and Intermittent Fasting really does wonders for your body. If you haven't lost any weight, not to fear. Your body is still adjusting.

Track and record your meals, your meal times, your exercise, and your experience during the first 10 days of this challenge!

Intermediate Intermittent Fasting

Day 11

This intermediate section is all about both reducing your eating windows and reducing your meals from three down to two, plus getting used to longer fasts and keeping up an exercise regimen, too. Since your body is adjusting to a fasting schedule, don't overdo it on your workouts. Start out with light exercise for about 20 minutes a day, then gently increase as the days go by.

Today, you're going to drop back from a 9 hour eating window to an 8 hour eating window. You'll still eat your three meals today, but you might need to adjust the times. You can also adjust the calorie percentages, like the different meal plan templates in Chapter 4. Adjust your meal plan as well. How is your new eating window time? It it is working out, great! After fasting for ten days, your body does start to change!

Track and record your new eating window, meal times, what you ate, your exercise, and your fasting experience.

Day 12

The 8 hour eating window / 16 hour fasting time is one of the most popular Intermittent Fasting schedules. It's especially great for women, since you get a lot of calories in a short period of time, but your body doesn't start to operate like it's a time of true scarcity.

Repeat your 8 hour eating window today. You fasted for 16 hours between yesterday and today. Eat your meals at their scheduled times.

Track and record what you ate and any exercise, too.

Day 13

Day 13 is just a repeat of yesterday: eating for 8 hours and fasting for 16 hours. As a general reminder, get plenty of water during fasting periods. You can increase your exercise up to 30 minutes if you want, but not if you are feeling weak or struggling with this eating routine. Allow your body plenty of time to adjust.

Track and record what you eat, how you feel, and any exercise.

Day 14

Congrats – you've reached the end of your second week Intermittent Fasting! You went from a 9-hour eating window to an 8-hour eating window, and are now fasting for 16 hours within each 24-hour cycle. That's extra hours your body spends pulling fuel sources from existing fat cells rather than any incoming nutrients.

It's time to assess the week. How did you do on increasing your Intermittent Fasting? Was it easy to adjust to 8 hours of eating? Have you been tracking everything each day? Weigh yourself today as well – and take a picture. How is your weight loss going?

Today, you will continue on your 8 hour eating window, just like yesterday. Eat your meals at their scheduled time. By now, you are really getting the hang of Intermittent Fasting. Track and record everything, too.

Day 15

Day 15 starts with an even smaller eating window – this one is just 7 hours. That means you'll be fasting for 17 hours within each 24 hour cycle. As you drop one more hour from eating, readjust both your meal plan and your meal times, too. We'll repeat this for several days, so make sure it's a time you're comfortable with. Get plenty of water during fasting periods. You can do your exercise today, too, if you want.

Dropping from 8 hours down to 7 hours started producing much more dramatic weight loss results for me. That result might be typical for you as well. Track and record your new eating window, your new meal times, and how you're doing. As a brief reminder, you have flexibility with your new eating windows, too.

Day 16

Today is a repeat of yesterday, with your 7 hours of eating and 17 hours of fasting. You fasted for the longest period of yet between yesterday and today, so how did that go? Slowly reintroduce your exercising again today, if you gave yourself a day off yesterday.

Track and record what you ate today.

Day 17

Today is the last day of the 7 hour eating window / 17 hour fasting times, so enjoy it! We're going to drop down to just a 6 hour eating window tomorrow. If you want to do anything to prepare for that shorter eating window, then do it today. Those preparations might include changing your meal times, cutting down from three meals to two, or even trying the one meal a day (OMAD) fasting.

Within your 7 hour eating window today, get all of your calories in before the time is up. Track and record everything that you ate, what you experienced, and any other notes.

Day 18

We're going to drop one more hour off of our Intermittent Fasting schedule today and go down to the 6 hour eating window / 18 hour fasting time. Together with the 8 hour eating window, this is the most common schedule for Intermittent Fasters. Those who do like this schedule usually eat just two meals a day, because the 6 hour time frame is so short. If you do that, then you will need to adjust your meal plan, your calorie percentages, and your meal times accordingly. Check out the two meal a day sample templates in Chapter 4 for exactly how to do this.

Is it okay to stick with an 8 hour or 7 hour eating window instead? Absolutely. Only go down to 6 hours if you feel comfortable with it. This eating window produces great results. You're encouraged to at least try it! Especially when you combine it with exercise. The weight starts to come off faster and faster.

So, eat your meals at your new meal times. Then track and record what you ate and when.

Day 19

We're going to stick with the 6 hour eating window / 18 hour fasting schedule today. How did last night's 18 hour fast go? Were you very hungry when you got up today, or has your body adjusted to fasting? Make any tweaks or changes if necessary. It's also okay to take a break from fasting if you're not feeling well.

However, if you are doing well, then I encourage you to also keep up with your exercise program. Don't forget to track and record what you ate at your meal times.

Day 20

So, you got through the second phase of Intermittent Fasting! You started out with an 8 hour eating window, then dropped down to 7, and are now at just 6 hours per day, with 18 hours of straight fasting. That's quite an accomplishment. You've probably also dropped down to just two meals a day and increased your calorie percentages for those meals. All those extra hours are when your body is using fat sources from your cells as energy, rather than relying on new foods that you're eating. Oh, and when you've added an exercise regimen to it, that is a recipe for success.

It's time to assess the past ten days. How have you been doing? Weigh yourself to see if you've lost more weight. You will start to feel big changes in your body.

In the next ten days, we will go into more advanced fasting, including a 24-hour fast and eating just OMAD (one meal a day).

As for today, just continue with your 6 hour eating window / 18 hour fasting. Track and record what you ate today, too.

Advanced Intermittent Fasting

Day 21

You are going to continue with your 6 hour eating window / 18 hour fasting schedule today. Also, you will want to read over the next ten days and prepare your meal plan accordingly for the 24-hour fast on Day 23 and the OMAD (one meal a day) days as well. After you have prepared your meal plan, today would be the ideal time to create your grocery list and shop for the ingredients you'll need.

As for today, just track and record what you ate, when your mealtimes are, and any exercise routine.

Day 22

Today is all about preparing for tomorrow's 24 hour fast. It's imperative that you make sure to eat all of your calories within your 6 hour window today. Also, abstain from exercising today, tomorrow, and on Day 24, to give your muscles a chance to fully rest. Eat your regular 6 hour eating window today, and begin your fast at the normal time.

Day 23

Today is your first 24 hour Intermittent Fasting day! Count 24 hours from the end of yesterday's eating window. Don't eat any calories throughout the entire time of fasting. For example, if your 6-hour eating window ended at 6:00 pm yesterday, you're not to eat anything until 6:00 pm today.

During your fast, you're allowed to have water. Don't exercise other than a very light walk if you want to do so.

When you do break your fast, do so gently. Eat a meal that has a good healthy protein and mineral rich foods like dark greens, avocados, nuts, and olives. Don't worry about eating your entire calorie percentage for the day. Just stop all eating about two hours before bed-time.

Track and record your 24-hour fast experience, including the meal to break your fast.

Day 24

How did yesterday's fast go? Today, you will return to the normal 6 hour eating window at the exact same times you had it on Day 22. Eat your normal calories like you would on any other day, and eat your meals at the same times as Day 22. Hydrate yourself with plenty of water, since that will also help flush out toxins and get your skin glowing. Help your body refuel from the fast by eating healthy today. Don't worry about getting any exercise today. You can if you want to!

Track and record your meals today.

Day 25

Today, you will repeat your regular 6 hour eating window / 18 hour fasting time. Eat the same number of meals at the same times that you were eating on Day 21. Also today, you will add back in the exercise routine that you have been on. Try for 30 minutes to get your heart rate up. You can do any exercise that you want.

Track and record your meals, the times, and your exercise.

Day 26

Tomorrow is when we are going to try OMAD (one meal a day), so today is about preparing for that. Eat your normal 6 hour eating window with the normal meal times, add exercise, track what you eat, and record your experience. You might want to prepare your singular meal recipes for tomorrow ahead of time.

Day 27

Today is a day to try the advanced fasting technique of OMAD. Choose a 60-minute free period of time today, and eat all of your calories within that 60 minute sitting. It's similar to having a large holiday meal! Don't overstuff yourself, but do get all of your calories in at once. Once the 60 minutes are over, that is when your eating window is done. You will fast until tomorrow, with nothing to consume except water.

Track what you ate today, when, and how you like eating one meal a day. It's definitely an interesting concept to try eating all of your calories just once a day.

Day 28

Repeat your one meal a day from yesterday, eating all of your calories within 60 minutes. Have your single meal at the same time you ate the one meal yesterday, to give your body the complete benefits of a 23-hour fasting time. Don't forget to exercise today, too.

Track and record what you ate and when.

Day 29

Today is a third day to try eating just one meal a day. Do you like it, or do you prefer longer eating windows? Consume all of your daily calories in just one meal. That leaves the rest of the day to fill with all of your activities! You can add in your exercise regimen as well today.

Track and record your one meal, when you ate it, what you had, and how you exercised.

Day 30

Wow, congratulations! You have reached the end of the intense 30 Day Intermittent Fasting Challenge. You got through several days of a short 6 hour eating window, the 24 hour fast on Day 23, and a couple of days of just trying the famous OMAD option! It's been quite the month to start from a 10 hour eating window on Day 1 and then get all the way here. So, congrats again on your success.

Time to weigh yourself again! How much weight have you lost? The successful combination of healthy eating, Intermittent Fasting, and regular exercise can really get you the results that you're looking for. Were you able to hit a goal weight loss? Did you stick with the Intermittent Fasting throughout the month? Even if you just decided to stay with the 8-hour eating window, that's still spending 112 hours a week fasting. It makes such a difference.

No matter how your experience went, you should celebrate! Show off your progress by posting those cool "before" and "after" photos of yourself. Look back over your food diary entries you've kept for the past thirty days. You can share those, too. Post your progress. You never know who you'll inspire – maybe even yourself!

What Works Best For You

The 30 Day Challenge is designed to give you a day by day account of how the Intermittent Fasting eating plans and lifestyle actually fit into a real woman's life.

Where do you take it from here?

Well, this 30 Day Challenge also introduced you to three main types of Intermittent Fasting:

1. 10, 9, 8, 7, or 6 hour eating windows with the appropriate fasting times
2. A longer 24-hour fast that could also be extended up to 36 or even 48 hours
3. Eating one meal a day within one hour and fasting the rest of the time

Whichever one you choose is that which works best with your lifestyle and your personal weight loss goals! Some women will do great on just shorter eating windows, and others will want to push themselves in order to try new things. Make this diet yours!

Thank you so much for going on this 30 Day Challenge and stretching your mindset about the link between when you're eating and when you're fasting! Are you ready for even more tips to help you? Then read on to the next chapter.

Chapter 9:
Get the Most Out of Your
Intermittent Fasting

Going through the 30 Day Challenge in the previous chapter has certainly given you an amazing foundation for incorporating any type of Intermittent Fasting into your life.

Now, you're going to boost up and derive the most amount of benefits from staying on Intermittent Fasting!

Cleaning Up With Autophagy

We're constantly learning new things about how our body's cells work. Since the dieting industry is such an enormous business, scientists study exactly how nutrients impact our body, how our body processes nutrients, and the link between nutrition and fuel.

One scientist studies a revolutionary cellular process that's the scientific proof behind why Intermittent Fasting works. Japanese cell biologist Yoshinori Ohsumi discovered this process, which is called autophagy. His work was such a breakthrough, he won the 2016 Nobel Prize in Physiology or Medicine.

What's autophagy – and what does it have to do with Intermittent Fasting?

Autophagy comes from the Greek words for "self-devouring." Sounds a bit gruesome, but it is a natural process that your cells go through all the time. In essence, autophagy is cellular spring cleaning. Your cell can actually disassemble its own unnecessary or non-functioning components and recycle those components. Autophagy is activated when you fast, because it is a natural response to the lack of incoming sufficient fuel sources: good fats, proteins, carbohydrates, or sugars.

Cells that perform autophagy are actually removing their own harmful and toxic components. Those components are responsible for so many bad things that happen to your body as you age, including:

- Skin damage, like wrinkles and sagging skin
- Failing eyesight and hearing
- Memory problems
- Loss of energy
- Increasing aches and pains
- A more sluggish metabolism
- Continual weight gain or stagnant weight that won't come off

The cellular components causing all of these issues are just like old junky clutter hanging on inside your cells. But when you are on the Keto Diet and Intermittent Fasting at the same time, your cells get the message that it is time to clean out all that stuff. It's removed as waste or toxins and some parts are recycled to make your cells run better, faster, more efficient, and ultimately healthier for you. The result is that you feel better, look better, and actually slow down the aging process!

But that's the power of autophagy!

You can absolutely trigger autophagy by just fasting on a regular diet that includes higher carbohydrates. But ultimately, it's the combination of Intermittent Fasting and the high fat fuel source on the Ketogenic Diet that really causes your cells to internally clean house!

That's right, ladies – Intermittent Fasting can be a key to slowing down the aging process.

That's because the autophagy from Intermittent Fasting leads to amazing changes at the cellular level.

Speed Up Cell Repair and Regeneration

You are made up of trillions of cells that are continuously going through their life cycles. As time goes on and you age, it's harder to replace cells, repair cells, and regenerate cells. You see it as aging – the loss of energy, being more susceptible to illness, getting creaky joints and arthritis, failing eyesight, hearing loss, and a host of other symptoms.

But you can definitely help turn back the clock by Intermittently Fasting! Especially when combined with a low carb, high (good) fat diet, those processes definitely increase your stem cell production, and stem cells can magically morph into any cell your body needs.

So, those great stem cells can now be used to keep you feeling fit and younger, even down to the cellular level. Just because you can't see it, though, doesn't mean you can't feel it! You definitely will.

Intermittent Fasting Increases HGH

What's HGH (human growth hormone), and why is it a good thing that Intermittent Fasting increases it? Just like other well known hormones such as your estrogen, HGH is a natural substance. It's produced by your pituitary gland and goes straight to your liver for metabolism. HGH is a 'monitoring' hormone that affects many processes in your body, including:

- Muscle and bone growth
- Sugar and fat metabolism
- Body fluids
- Overall body composition
- Cell regeneration and reproduction
- Slowing down aging
- Recovering from both disease and injury

When you don't have enough HGH, then that increases body fat, a lower lean body mass, and even decreased bone mass. In short, it's a good thing when HGH is increased. If you fast for just a 24 hour period, you can potentially increase your HGH production naturally by 1300%. That's plenty to give you all those above benefits all their own.

The HGH production is also triggered by the state of ketosis in your body, which I'll go into detail in the next chapter.

Give Yourself an Energy Boost-Up

Intermittent Fasting does NOT decrease your energy – it actually increases it!

But this is another myth that seems like it should be true. After all, the less we eat, the less energetic we feel, right? But it doesn't make sense from a historical perspective.

Let's say it's 30,000 years ago, and a human hasn't eaten for a single day. If that person's metabolism decreased after just one day of fasting, then they wouldn't have any energy to go out to hunt or gather more food! After a second day, supposedly that person would be even weaker. If energy continually was lost after fasting, our species would not have survived. We needed energy even after fasting to go out and hunt more food.

So, when you're fasting, your metabolism actually goes up. You're burning more stored fat as fuel, and that increases your metabolism. It also means your personal energy supply doesn't run out. As long as you've got plenty of stored fat for your liver to turn into ketones for fuel, your metabolism and energy levels will be just fine!

The Benefits of Exercise

I've touched a bit on exercising in Chapter 6, when talking about how to start with a simple exercise regimen. If you haven't already done so, go back and read that section. It will give you one of the easiest and simplest step by step routines towards incorporating exercise into your lifestyle and combining it with an Intermittent Fasting eating routine.

You can definitely lose weight just by Intermittent Fasting. Simply follow the 30 Day Challenge in the previous chapter to find your ideal eating window amount of time and then fast the rest of the time.

But how would you like to boost up your weight loss into that kind of magical territory that you see online in Instagram pictures, Facebook posts, and magazine stories? You know, the kinds where you see women have lost forty, fifty, sixty, or even a hundred pounds in less than a year?

You will see the common denominator for those women was that they added exercise to their Intermittent Fasting and healthy eating. It really kickstarts your body into a state of significant weight loss!

Would you like to feel not just leaner, but stronger, too? Then I highly suggest adding some mild weight training to your exercise program. I use light kettlebells to help build up my muscles and burn even more fat from my adipose cells. You actually gain muscle when you fast, which is why it's become very popular with men who want to bulk up! But even us girls can have an amazingly toned and well muscled body from combining weight training with Intermittent Fasting.

On the Fast Track

One last benefit that will really turbocharge your Intermittent Fasting? Combining it with the Keto Diet. This is another piece of the weight loss puzzle that thousands of women have had success with.

So, how do you do that? In the next chapter, we'll definitely go in depth into it!

Chapter 10:
The Keto Diet and Intermittent Fasting

By now, you've probably heard of the Ketogenic Diet, nicknamed the Keto Diet for short. This is a very powerful and some say life-changing eating plan. It has some restrictions, so I only recommend it for those women who have really gotten comfortable with your Intermittent Fasting eating windows, eating healthier, and adding your own exercise regimen.

But once you have, then get ready for some miraculous body transformations. The Keto Diet is a diet of extremes. We're going to take the 'balanced diet' idea and completely throw it out!

The Keto Diet is a very high (good) fat, very low carb eating plan. We're talking over 100 grams of fat and less than 30 grams of carbohydrates per day. But it's these kinds of extremes that will get you massive results.

All About Ketosis

The Keto Diet actually changes your body's metabolic processes from one that mostly runs on glucose and glycogen from carbohydrates to one that primarily runs on ketones that come from those fat cells processed in your liver. When you are using ketones as your number one fuel, you're said to be in ketosis.

Ketosis is not a singular bodily function, but rather a series of processes that activate certain cells to stop doing things they were before and start doing new things.

Take a look at the whole process in action:

You Eat Good Fats

|

Fats Enter the Stomach

|

Liver Breaks Down Fats For Energy (Beta-Oxidation)

|

Liver Produces Ketones

|

Ketones Used As Fuel

|

Liver Also Uses Stored Fat to Make Ketones

Ketones Used As Fuel

Say, look at that! We're back to using your stored fat as fuel, which is exactly what we want. You want to be in a state of ketosis while you're Intermittently Fasting in order to gain the maximum benefits from both.

How can you tell you're in ketosis? You will need to purchase a special monitor that can test your urine, breath, or blood to be sure. Your reading tells you exactly how many ketones your liver is producing for fuel. These monitors can be purchased online or at a store like Amazon or Walmart.

When you're just starting out on the diet, check for ketosis every day. Once you are in ketosis and you get a feel for that metabolic state in your body, then you can measure your ketones every three or four days. If you eat too many carbohydrate foods, you could knock yourself out of ketosis.

The Keto Macros

Remember how I talked at length about Fats, Proteins, and Carbohydrates back in Chapters 3 and 4? That's because in the Keto Diet world, those three are called Macronutrients. These 'Macros' form the basis for the Keto Diet and are the main thing you track each and every day. On the Keto Diet, calories matter, but not as much as getting the right amount of your Macros.

I suggested back in Chapter 4 that you should eat healthy carbohydrates and grain foods that have a lot of fiber. You can eat up to 30% carbohydrates on some of the meal plan templates.

But your Macros on a Ketogenic Diet are vastly different.

You should be consuming 70% of your daily calories from those good fat sources, 19% of your proteins from natural animal and plant sources, and 5% - 8% of your carbohydrates from healthy sources.

For a woman's Macro requirements, it looks like this:

70% FATS – 19% PROTEINS – 5% CARBOHYDRATES

These are the Macros that you should track, and the proper percentages that you need in order to get into ketosis and stay in that metabolic state.

There are many online Ketogenic Macro calculators, and I encourage you to calculate your exact Macro percentages. They change depending on many factors in your physicality, including your height, weight, current age, and BMI.

As a general guideline when reading about the contents of these Macros on a food label, you should look for these quantities:

167g FATS – 100g PROTEINS – 25g CARBOHYDRATES

That adds up to 292 total grams of food per day. These are the Macros that you should be tracking each day that you're on the Ketogenic Diet.

These are the daily amounts that will kick your body into a ketosis state and start burning massive amounts of stored fat.

Keto Approved Foods

How are you supposed to eat nearly 170 grams of fat per day and yet far less than 30 grams of carbohydrates per day?

By sticking to the Keto Diet approved foods list! Below, I've put together the top 10 most common Ketogenic approved foods. This is an excellent base to get you started on the road towards changing your diet to the Keto one.

Produce:

1. Avocados
2. Lemons
3. Onions
4. Green Bell Peppers
5. Button Mushrooms
6. Romaine Lettuce
7. Fresh Spinach
8. Kale
9. Broccoli
10. Cauliflower

Meat & Seafood:

1. Steak (Flank and Skirt)
2. Ground Beef
3. Bacon
4. Shrimp
5. Cod Fillets

6. Boneless Chicken Breasts / Thighs
7. Pork Chops
8. Salami
9. Prosciutto
10. Lamb

Eggs & Dairy:

1. Eggs
2. High Quality Grass-Fed Butter
3. Heavy Cream
4. Cheddar Cheese
5. Mozzarella Cheese
6. Parmesan Cheese
7. Cream Cheese
8. Sour Cream
9. Goat Cheese
10. Plain Greek Yogurt

Herbs & Spices:

1. Salt
2. Pepper
3. Fresh Garlic Cloves
4. Fresh Herbs (parsley, cilantro, dill, etc.)
5. Dried Italian Herbs
6. Cinnamon
7. Thyme
8. Chili Powder
9. Onion Powder
10. Ginger

Oils & Condiments:

1. Olive Oil
2. Coconut Oil
3. Sesame Oil
4. Flavored Oils

5. Mayonnaise
6. Dijon Mustard
7. Fish Sauce
8. Hot Sauce
9. Lemon Juice
10. Soy Sauce

Nuts & Seeds:

1. Macadamia Nuts
2. Pecans
3. Walnuts
4. Almonds
5. Nut Butters
6. Pumpkin Seeds
7. Sunflower Seeds
8. Sesame Seeds
9. Ground Flax Seeds
10. Chia Seeds

Baking & Broths:

1. Almond Flour
2. Coconut Flour
3. Cocoa Powder
4. Baking Powder
5. Vanilla Extract
6. Sugar-Free Dark Chocolate
7. Stevia
8. Unsweetened Almond Milk
9. Chicken Broth
10. Beef Broth

Other:

1. MCT Oil
2. Green Olives
3. Black Coffee

4. Black or Green Teas
5. Wine
6. Dill Pickles
7. Canned Tomatoes
8. Full Fat Coconut Milk
9. Curry Pastes (red, green, yellow)
10. Psyllium Husk Powder

Those are the most essential eighty ingredients! There's plenty here to get you started. If you're having trouble meeting such a high fat requirement throughout your eating window, then take a look at the following foods and their high fat percentages:

1. Butter – 100% fat
2. Olive Oil – 100% fat
3. MCT Oil – 100% fat
4. Heavy Cream – 95% fat
5. Green Olives – 88% fat
6. Macadamia Nuts – 88% fat
7. Cream Cheese – 88% fat
8. Sour Cream – 86% fat
9. Coconut Cream – 86% fat
10. Walnuts – 84% fat
11. Brazil Nuts – 84% fat
12. Almond Butter – 79% fat
13. Avocado – 77% fat

All of these foods are not only delicious, they can help you meet those fat gram requirements.

Just like in the 30 Day Intermittent Fasting Challenge chapter in this book, you want to be diligent about tracking your Macros each and every day. When you're on the Keto Diet, it's largely about the numbers. Eat as many good fats as you can to hit that high level required, keep your healthy protein intake to a medium level, and slash that carbohydrate number down to one that is very small.

If you have any questions about putting together meals from these ingredients and finding even more ingredients that are Keto approved, I suggest you buy a specific Keto book! That will go into so much more detail.

The Keto Diet and Intermittent Fasting

Why do Intermittent Fasting and the Keto Diet work so well together?

That's because Intermittent Fasting helps your body get into ketosis faster and helps maintain that metabolic state even longer than if you weren't fasting.

What this means, is that you can supercharge the benefits that you get from Intermittent Fasting. You will go into ketosis quickly, and also begin burning the fat from your cells that much sooner.

Going Keto is the ultimate boost up for Intermittent Fasting.

Chapter 11:
Conclusion

Thank you so much for reading all the way down to this chapter! I've had a lot of fun putting this book together for you. I've shared with you my personal story, my own tips and tricks, and I've also shown you that I'm a woman just like you who is looking for the same things as you are:

A healthy, natural, and pretty effortless way

to reach and stay at my goal weight.

When I first stumbled across Intermittent Fasting, I was skeptical and I messed it up. It's only when I really began to take it seriously and find ways to make it work in my real life (house, husband, kids, job, and all!) that I was finally able to reach that goal weight number.

Intermittent Fasting and You

Now it's your turn to take this book with you on your own Intermittent Fasting journey. It won't look like mine, although you'll find my advice so helpful and useful. But your journey will be unique. You may have a different eating window than me. You have a different life than me.

That's why I urge you to take Intermittent Fasting seriously and spend the time to make it your own. See it as a great challenge to incorporate it into your existing life. This isn't an eating plan that's only for celebrities, women in warm climates, women who are really well-off or wealthy, women who do have kids or don't have kids, or any other kind of woman!

This is an eating plan for you. It's so flexible that it fits every woman. Think of it like finding that absolute perfect fitting outfit. It's the perfect color, perfect fabric, perfect fit, it shows off what you want to show off, it conceals what you want to conceal, it's comfortable, and it even has decent pockets! Now that really would be the perfect outfit, right?

Intermittent Fasting is like that. It's great for you, because you make it your own.

A Calendar and a Calculator

If you really want to know the secrets to dieting success, let me point you to two very simple, very inexpensive office tools:

- A calendar
- A calculator

Your Intermittent Fasting lifestyle is intricately connected to your calendar days. It is a schedule as much as it is an eating plan. You schedule your eating windows, you schedule your fasting times, and you schedule in exercising, too.

Eating on the Intermittent Fasting way also requires a calculator to stay within your Macro percentages during your meal times in your eating windows. You are calculating the calories that you eat as well. If you decide to try the Ketogenic Diet in conjunction with Intermittent Fasting, you will be calculating and adding up your Macros each day, too.

So, that's it – just a calendar and a calculator are your primary weight loss tools. That's how I started, and that's an excellent place for you to get started, too.

How to Enjoy Intermittent Fasting

I don't know about you, but if something is not enjoyable for me, I just won't do it. I learned long ago that trying to force myself (different than getting out of my comfort zone) was just completely counter-productive.

Then, I discovered something. It happened while I was trying to get my kids to do chores. I realized that if I made it enjoyable in any way – singing, make it a game, playing – then they happily responded and helped do their chores.

Well, even though I'm a mom and an adult, I'm still just a big kid. I knew I had to make Intermittent Fasting enjoyable for me in some way as well. The same goes for you. When you make this eating plan enjoyable, it stops being about work and starts being more about a great part of your life. You might think I'm a little nuts, but I actually look forward to fasting!

So, how can you enjoy Intermittent Fasting and have a great time doing it? Here are things I've done myself:

- Play around with flavors and recipes in the kitchen. I just love trying new dishes, expanding my palate, and discovering a new spice, fruit, vegetable, herb, or grain I've never tried before. With online choices from Amazon, you can buy all kinds of wonderful ingredients.
- Use your fasting times to do something fun for yourself that doesn't involve food. I only eat twice a day, so I am able to squeeze in some extra time to do stuff I love to do.
- Share your fasting story with friends. I love to text my girlfriends about my latest fasting experience. We cheer each other on. It's a lot of fun.

I just see my eating windows and fasting times as two different facets of the same thing – an eating plan that I can enjoy because it gets me results. Plus, I have fun with it along the way, too.

Future You Will Thank Today You

You can be on the Intermittent Fasting plan for as long as you like.

Think about how you'll feel two months, two years, two decades from now. Today really only is temporary. Think of how quickly the last two months have gone. It just flies by.

There are so many perks to this. I mean, have you ever kept your bigger clothes from season to season because you thought you might need them in the future? What if the future you is the same size for months at a time?

You can use Intermittent Fasting to obtain your goal weight and to stay there for months or even years at a time.

Happy Feelings, Healthy Body

Your happiness is tied to how you feel in your own skin. Your Intermittent Fasting success story is waiting for you to write it. When I started writing this book, I first outlined what I wanted to say, and then I spent many hours writing the words for you to read them. Your weight loss journey will be just like that.

You will spend time reading about Intermittent Fasting, just like you've done in this book, and then you will follow the 30 Day Challenge day by day towards losing the weight. That alone will give you an amazing variety of eating windows and fasting times.

Life is a wild ride, girl! Isn't it? It has its ups, downs, times when you're steadily going forward, and times when it feels like time has stopped and maybe you are even going backward.

You need an eating plan that can keep up with all of these crazy changes. You need to give Intermittent Fasting a try.

You'll feel better, and you'll have a healthier body, too. It's for yourself, for your family, for your friends, and for your own future, too. Fasting is your friend!

So we have reached this point where I hope to say that it is just a temporary good bye. I hope to see you in my other books focused on health, diet and nutrition.

Before you go though, could you do me a favor?

116

Please let us know what is the 1 or 2 things you picked up that is of value to you in this book and please share it as a review on amazon. This will be super helpful to others and also to let others know what you have learnt!

Thank you so so much !

Made in the USA
San Bernardino, CA
16 May 2019